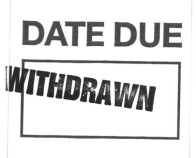

FREUD
VS.
GOD

How Psychiatry Lost Its Soul & Christianity Lost Its Mind

DAN BLAZER

InterVarsity Press
Downers Grove, Illinois

InterVarsity Press
P.O. Box 1400, Downers Grove, IL 60515
World Wide Web: www.ivpress.com
E-mail: mail@ivpress.com

InterVarsity Press® is the book-publishing division of InterVarsity Christian Fellowship/USA®, a student movement
active on campus at hundreds of universities, colleges and schools of nursing in the United States of America, and a
member movement of the International Fellowship of Evangelical Students. For information about local and
regional activities, write Public Relations Dept., InterVarsity Christian Fellowship/USA, 6400 Schroeder Rd., P.O.
Box 7895, Madison, WI 53707-7895.

ISBN 0-8308-1547-3

Printed in the United States of America ∞

Library of Congress Cataloging-in-Publication Data

Blazer, Dan G. (Dan German), 1944-
  Freud vs. God : how psychiatry lost its soul and Christianity lost
its mind / Dan Blazer.
    p.   cm.
  Includes bibliographical references.
  ISBN 0-8308-1547-3 (alk. paper)
  1. Psychiatry and religion.   2. Christianity—Psychology.
3. Psychotherapy—Religious aspects—Christianity.   I. Title.
  RC455.4.R4B56   1998
  261.5'15—dc21   *97-46382*
                                                                        CIP

21	20	19	18	17	16	15	14	13	12	11	10	9	8	7	6	5	4	3	2	1
16	15	14	13	12	11	10	09	08	07	06	05	04	03	02	01	00	99	98		

To
Bill Wilson
who believes passionately,
debates forcefully
and cares unceasingly
for the mentally ill

Acknowledgments

Many persons contributed to this volume. Yet none but I make the argument. To each I give credit for assisting me to formulate my argument, yet none can be blamed for my conclusions.

Ross Thomson, at one of our periodic Saturday-morning philosophical discussions, kindled the spark to begin this project. Stanley Haucrwas helped me shape my arguments and challenged me when I needed to be challenged. In addition, he always suggested one more book or paper to read. Keith Meador, Judy and Richard Hays, Bailey Forrest, Jerry Sprague and Bobbi Hendrix each read portions of the manuscript and provided me with critical feedback.

I cannot overestimate the excellent work of Rachel Toor. Rachel helped me find my genre, the essay, as the most comfortable means for making my argument and encouraged me to "put more of" myself into this book, which rendered the task a joy. Lavon Perkins patiently typed many drafts of the manuscript. Her pleasant and accommodating personality, coupled with her deep faith, was an inspiration throughout the months of preparation.

I wish to thank Rodney Clapp of IVP for both his encouragement and his thoughtful reading of the manuscript.

Finally, I acknowledge those who make my life worth living—Sherrill, Trey and Tasha. Not only have they supported me in my secular career, they are soul mates with me on our sacred journey.

Introduction: Christian and Psychiatrist

I am a Christian who practices psychiatry. It is a comfortable life, a *disturbingly* comfortable life. Something is missing.

As a fundamentalist, evangelical Christian physician entering psychiatric training, I prepared for a battle and an opportunity that never occurred. I feared that mentoring psychiatrists would attempt to retell my life story and shape my beliefs such that I would no longer accept the faith of my heritage. A psychiatrist would reach deep inside me and steal my good Father in heaven. No such battle occurred. I also wanted to help bridge the gap between psychiatry and evangelical Christianity. In retrospect, the drive to bridge that gap appeared unnecessary for both psychiatrists and Christians.

In the twenty-five years during which I have studied and practiced psychiatry, I have witnessed a dramatic and rapid, but often unrecognized, evolution in the approach of psychiatrists and Christians to the emotionally disturbed. This evolution, grounded in influences from earlier in the twentieth century, has profoundly restructured the conversation between psychiatry and Christianity, especially evangelical Christianity. I write this book to bring to light what I believe is missing from the current conversation.

During the first half of the twentieth century, psychiatrists, more than other physicians, were preoccupied with religion, and especially Christianity. This preoccupation, as illustrated in the writings of Sigmund Freud, C. G. Jung and others, first attracted me to psychiatry as a medical specialty, for I found their writings addressing the needs of persons in relationships rather than as conglomerates of isolated parts such as the gall bladder and heart. Christians, likewise, were intrigued by psychological explorations of their individual beliefs, especially beliefs associated with sin, and psychological theories that both informed the religious experience and provided practical guidelines for pastoral care. Within my faith community, while I attended medical school, pastors and other church leaders were attempting to combine biblical principles with psychological insights to help persons within the community who were experiencing emotional suffering.

The common interests of psychiatrists and Christians derived naturally from the recognition that psychiatric illness was at once brain dysfunction, psychological conflict and spiritual crisis. These common interests led initially to meaningful conversations and later heated debates between psychiatrists and Christians. I could not walk into my faith community or into the hospital where I trained in psychiatry without feeling the tension of the debates. I was an outsider in both communities: the psychiatrists thought I should commit myself to psychiatry, and the Christians thought I should commit myself to Christianity—but neither side thought I could or should commit myself to both.

The conversations between psychiatry and Christianity peaked less than fifty years ago and were often framed as the "Freud versus God debate." "Freud versus God" has, from the beginning, been a metaphor for the tension between psychoanalytic theory and Christian theology, two different worldviews. Both psychiatrists and Christian theologians engaged honestly and intelligently the angst experienced by modern humankind.

In the 1990s, however, psychiatrists and Christians (in particular evangelical Christians) seem to have reached a comfortable rapprochement. The conversation is subdued, and the debate has virtually ended. I feel comfortable and unchallenged in both communities, more secure but much less stimulated. And I believe that the task of bridging the gap was scarcely begun before it was prematurely ended.

A Conversation

The conversation between psychiatry and Christianity is of personal and professional interest to me. My roots are in fundamentalist, evangelical Christianity and academic psychiatry. My motivation for writing this book is to review and reflect on why the conversations of only a few decades ago have disappeared.

Psychiatry and Christianity have never experienced better superficial relations. Each has accommodated and, to some degree, assimilated the other. The tension between them, which should stimulate advances in our understanding of the deepest emotional pains, has given way to a comfortable segmentation of the brain from the soul.[1] Why? The existential pain and subjective experience of psychiatric illness are of little interest to modern psychiatrists. Meanwhile, the philosophical and theological implications of disorders of the brain and modern psychiatric therapies are of little interest to Christian theologians. As a result, in my opinion, psychiatry has lost its soul and Christianity has lost its mind.

Keeping Focus

Published literature about the relationship between psychiatry and religion would fill a small library. If I were to add the literature about the psychology of religion, the library would become very large indeed. I, personally, am fascinated by this literature but must necessarily omit from my present discussion many topics of interest to me and to others. In other words, I have no desire to write a comprehensive historical or theological/philosophical treatise. Rather, I present an argument in essay form, an argument drawn largely from my experience as a practicing academic psychiatrist and evangelical Christian. I believe my experience *can* be generalized to the dominant lack of conversation between psychiatrists and Christians. So I support my contentions with what I believe to be central rather than comprehensive references from this large library.

A book describing and reflecting on psychiatry and Christianity will necessarily omit significant historical and current themes in the interaction of religion and psychiatry. Psychiatry interacts with other religions besides Christianity: the Jewish faith, Islam and Eastern religions (which have, perhaps, focused more on the mind than other religions). Psychiatry practiced among Orthodox Jews or fundamentalist Muslims takes on a quite different quality from psychiatry practiced among Christians. For example, the psychiatrist in Saudi Arabia treating a strict Muslim suffering from alcohol abuse and dependence (it does happen!) has the full authority of the religious state and strong peer pressure from dominant social attitudes to reinforce a prescription of abstinence. Motivation to quit drinking derives more from external authority than from an appeal to the will of the alcoholic. Even the prescription of prayer assists the psychiatrist to reinforce the social sanctions of Islam, for the alcoholic Muslim prays with all other faithful Muslims.

In this discussion I pay less attention to the Catholic Church than Protestant groups, for I believe psychiatry's conversation with the Catholic Church is qualitatively different from that with Protestant Christianity. For example, the non-Catholic psychiatrist, whether religious or not, frequently cannot understand the strength and support the Catholic patient derives from the sacramental practices of the church. These practices may appear ritualistic and compulsive to the Protestant and therefore may quickly be dismissed as unhealthy.

Also, I do not explore significant variants from mainline and evangelical Protestant Christianity. The African-American church, for example, has a particular interest in the relevance of faith to emotional as well as social suffering. African-Americans are much less likely than whites to use psychiatric services, and the number of African-American psychiatrists remains appallingly small. If psychiatrists in general underestimate the potential support of the church for persons experiencing severe emotional problems, then they certainly underestimate the support and central role of the black church in the life of the African-American community. The church has become the point from which both spiritual and political power extends throughout the African-American community. Black church leaders are therefore not only advantageous but frequently necessary collaborators in treating problems such as drug abuse. But in this book I focus rather on the relationship of my own faith tradition, evangelical Protestant Christianity, to psychiatry.

I do not focus on other mental health professions whose practitioners are often concerned with emotional suffering and an approach to it based on their religious beliefs. These include psychologists, social workers, physicians other than psychiatrists, and nurses. I do not review in depth the discussions about mind and brain in light of recent discoveries about brain function—a discussion carried on by a few philosophers, theologians and psychologists. Psychology, as a discipline, has been more engaged in discussion of mind and soul than psychiatry. Associations such as the Association for Religious and Value Issues in Counseling and the Christian Association for Psychological Studies are dominated by psychologists, not psychiatrists. A strong division of the American Psychological Association (Division 36) is devoted to the study of the psychology of religion. In addition, a movement has evolved over many years, even centuries, to integrate psychology and theology/religion. In contrast, psychiatry, especially in recent years, has deviated from the task of interpretation even in the wake of greater accommodation.

So I write from the perspective of my own profession—psychiatry. Even so, my perspective will appear foreign to non-Christian psychiatrists and, to some extent, mainline Protestants. The sheer numbers of evangelical Christians, not to mention the political influence of the so-called Religious Right render my perspective relevant. Yet some may question whether I, or anyone else, can accurately represent evangelical thought. Diversity within the evangelical community is significant. For example, the members of my own faith tradition would take issue with my labeling myself as either an evangelical or as a Protestant. I am a member of the Church of Christ, noninstrumental variety. We typically describe ourselves as members of the restoration movement—that is, we are attempting to rescue Christianity from historical influences, whether Catholic, Protestant *or evangelical,* and restore the one true church of the first century of the Christian era. Even so, for the purposes of this book I believe I speak from the perspective of tens of millions among the evangelical ranks.

Two Forces

The story I tell is a story of two forces dominating the 1990s, that is, the rise of the evangelical Christian counseling industry and neuropsychiatry. I am not a philosopher. I am a practicing psychiatrist who treats Christians suffering from psychiatric illnesses and who examines theory in light of that practice. Yet both perceived needs of patients and responses by psychiatrists are shaped by forces that, I believe, are external to psychiatric theory and Christian theology and often not recognized.

For example, the desire for immediate relief from specific problems has driven Christians *and* psychiatrists to seek and prescribe quick solutions with little attention paid to the whole person. These forces have led Christian counselors and psychiatrists to ignore or deny the existential dimension of severe emotional suffering, neglect the life story of the sufferer, uncouple the life story from the Christian story, trivialize the Christian community as a source of healing, and superficially accommodate each other rather than engage in meaningful discourse. Psychiatrists and Christians have, in large part, drugged or denied pain and suffering and deemphasized the importance of embedding the often-troubled stories of our individual lives within communal life.

Therefore I offer my readers a critique of psychiatrists and Christians as they work in parallel to relieve emotional suffering. I tell a story of a conversation once joined and now abandoned. I propose that when psychiatrists and Christians honestly reflect on severe emotional suffering, they cannot but engage in serious and meaningful dialogue, and perhaps tense but productive debate. As things stand, psychiatrists and Christians are carrying on superficial cocktail-party talk rather than sitting at the table of serious conversation. Perhaps psychiatrists and Christians alike could learn from the poet Rainer Maria Rilke in his *Letters to a Young Poet:*

> Whoever looks seriously at it [love and marriage] finds that it will not be possible to find any general rule resting in agreement. . . . The demands which the difficult work of love makes upon our development are more than life-size, and as beginners we are not up to them. But if we nevertheless hold out and take love upon us as *burden* and apprenticeship, instead of losing ourselves in all light and frivolous play, behind which people have hidden from the most earnest earnestness of their existence—then a little progress and an alleviation will perhaps be perceptible

to those who come long after us; that would be much.[2]
I do not expect psychiatrists and Christians to marry their views. Yet
psychiatrists and Christians are mutually engaged with many people suffering emotional distress. If we truly care about those we care for, we should
take upon ourselves the burden of the conversation and debate. Then we can
realistically expect that "little progress" in our own capabilities as caretak-
ers of persons with severe emotional problems.

My Story
I believe my own story provides an example of how quickly one can slip
into easy accommodation and avoid the burden of serious conversation. For
this reason I describe my initial fears of psychiatry, my unexpected but
readily accepted comfortable life as a psychiatrist and the nagging questions
presented to me by the patients with whom I have worked. These patients
have, in turn, forced me not only to engage in an internal conversation but
also to expose my conflicts and naked ignorance to others.

Writing this book is perhaps the most difficult task I have undertaken as
an academic psychiatrist. Yet it is a task that will bring me little credit as an
academician. I have already established my reputation and advanced far in
the academic ranks. This book will not be counted toward my academic
productivity, for it is not a product of rigorous scholarship. Rather, here I
attempt to explore and express concerns that plague me personally, not just
address an interesting intellectual question.

Work on this book has required me to take on another challenge, to cross
the boundary of my academic comfort zone. I have presented my ideas and
beliefs to professional theologians and to the very Christian counselors and
psychiatrists whom I criticize. In other words, I have broadened and
deepened my own relationships. This exposure has been stimulating, for it
has opened a new world of intellectual inquiry and pointed me to writings
that have addressed the very issues about which I have been concerned,
writings of which I had not been aware. Some of the most exciting and
challenging conversations of my career have come as a result of writing this
book. Yet these interrelations have exposed my ignorance of topics about
which I thought I knew something. I had become unaccustomed to being

told I was "uninformed," "amateur" and "lacking scholarship." I feel more like an undergraduate student than a professor when I write at the interface of psychiatry and religion. Yet I believe the effort is necessary to move me further along a path on which I could become stagnant. The path I have chosen is not the path I expected, nor the path expected of me.

I grew up in the buckle of the Bible Belt of the southern United States—Nashville, Tennessee. My family had been faithful, fundamentalist Christians for at least three generations on both sides, and my parents maintained that tradition. From my perspective as a child, the "fundamentals" began with the Bible as the infallible Word of God. To be saved from hell, I had to accept the Scriptures as the literal guide for my life, and because I was saved as a Christian, I was different. I was "set apart from the world," and some outward behaviors were involved in setting me apart. Three times a week I attended the fundamental Church of Christ. I did not smoke, drink or curse, and even during my teenage years, I tried to "set an example" to those around me of what it meant to be a Christian.

In retrospect, I recognize that my perception of being different also meant that I separated myself from theology, philosophy and most professions. I could not conceive of a future in an academic discipline. Even today I feel most at home in the Church of Christ, where I currently serve as an elder. It is true that during my lifetime my church family has changed, becoming more educated and less rigid. Yet neither I nor the Church of Christ has wandered far from our fundamental, simple and separatist roots.

I dreamed, as a teenager, of becoming a medical missionary so that I might combine my interest in healing the sick with my religious beliefs. The dream of being a doctor was a dream of serving, not a dream of exploring how the body or the mind works. I realized this dream, following graduation from medical school and internship, by spending two years as a missionary in Africa. Though I did not expect mission work in an underdeveloped country to be easy, I was comfortable with the idea of serving, for each day I expected to begin my work with the conviction that my work and faith were in concert. In what better way could a follower of Jesus Christ live the story of the "Great Physician" than to become a physical and spiritual minister to those in pain?

Yet while in medical school, before I went to Africa, I was derailed from my adolescent dream and attracted to psychiatric writings, especially the writings of Sigmund Freud. I realized that I didn't understand myself well, especially my puritanical, serious desire to serve, and perhaps to suffer. Freud suggested that I might be motivated by factors other than a simple faith in God and a desire to do his will. Yet Freud appeared anti-Christian, and his teachings dominated psychiatry at the time. Therefore I believed Christians should naturally be in conflict with psychiatrists. I found, however, that Freud spoke a language that appealed to my perception of the nature of humankind, a language of integration and relatedness. Not only were the biological and psychological to be considered in healing the emotions, but the cultural and the spiritual should be considered as well. Yet Freud went further. The neuropsychological and spiritual were the same. Freud appeared to speak of body and soul as one, not in conflict. To me, Freud was a doctor of the soul. I wanted to be a doctor who worked with patients in relation to others and to God.

I decided to enter psychiatric training upon completion of medical mission work. Friends and family believed I was being seduced toward a career that was not compatible with my faith. Yet the potential to heal painful emotions seemed, at the time, worth the internal struggle I would face as a Christian in secular psychiatry. I expected my beliefs to be challenged and my lifestyle to be perceived odd, if not prudish, by my psychiatric teachers and colleagues. When I entered psychiatric training in 1973, no psychiatrist, to my knowledge, was counted among the two million active members of the fundamentalist Churches of Christ. I could be a pioneer, struggling to resolve the conflict between psychiatry and fundamental Christianity, proving that one could be a faithful Christian and practice psychiatry. The practice (in contrast to the theory) of Freudian psychiatry did not appear that far removed from the practice of the Christian confessional. Growth through the miracle of dialogue was the foundation of both psychiatric therapy and Christian salvation. The mission I set for myself would be far more difficult than mission work in Africa. I would be challenged by my psychiatric colleagues from without and would struggle within to integrate psychiatry and Christianity.

I arrived at Duke University School of Medicine to train in psychiatry following my two years in Africa. What I found surprised me. I found a faculty member in psychiatry who was an evangelical Christian and expressed his beliefs in both his conversations and his practice. He even prayed with his patients! And he was no more or less isolated from mainstream psychiatry at Duke than anyone else. There was no mainstream! Among the faculty I found behaviorists, Freudian analysts, Jungian analysts, social psychiatrists and psychopharmacologists. Actually most of the faculty were eclectic, combining whatever therapies appeared to be effective. I suspect the department of psychiatry at Duke was unique compared to other psychiatry departments in the United States during the late 1960s and early 1970s, for no ideology predominated. Yet Duke was at the vanguard of what was to happen in psychiatry over the next few decades.

I was also surprised at my reception by Duke. Not only did I come from a conservative Christian background, I also came from a southern, state-supported medical school. I feared that not only my religious beliefs but also my lack of sophisticated education (even my southern accent) would isolate me from the academic community of psychiatrists. Nothing could have been further from reality during my years of training in psychiatry at Duke. I was accepted, mentored and even encouraged to pursue an academic, scholarly career.

I decided to pursue such a career, which I expected to crystallize the inherent conflict between psychiatry and Christianity for me. The window was social psychiatry (see chapter three), which was active at the time—the study of emotional suffering in the context of relations between the person and society. Society includes not only interpersonal relations but also the cultural and religious context in which the person lives. Surely when I explored the boundaries of knowledge in psychiatry, my religious beliefs would be challenged from without and within.

That challenge from without and struggle within never materialized. As a Christian, I have not been relegated to the periphery of psychiatry. Rather, I have worked at the very center of academic psychiatry. I have remained an active churchman, my beliefs have changed little, and frankly, I have carved out a comfortable life within my profession and within my faith community. My academic pursuits did not require me to explore the theological and philosophical conflicts between psychiatry and Christianity, much less struggle with them.

What happened? Why did the conflicts I expected never materialize? How can I treat the severely depressed in my office with an antidepressant medication and modern psychotherapy while at the same time teach about the reality of sin and the inevitability of emotional suffering each Sunday morning to a Bible school class?

Reopening the Conversation

During the early and mid-twentieth century, conversations did emerge between psychiatrists and Christian theologians comparing and integrating Freud's theory of the origins of emotional suffering with the Christian explanations of sin and spiritual growth. These conversations, however, did not, for the most part, reach the more conservative, evangelical Christian in the pew. A vague but strong perception that psychiatry was to be avoided by believing evangelical Christians emerged, often framed as the "Freud versus God" debate. Evangelical Christians were fearful of Freudian psychiatry and expressed little interest in dialogue. Among some psychiatrists, Christians who interpreted Scripture literally were belittled as emotionally immature, and their faith was dismissed rather than discussed in depth. So the conflict between psychiatry and conservative Christianity never gained momentum and has now largely disappeared.

I began my career as a psychiatrist at the very time when the so-called Freud versus God debate was fading to the background for both psychiatrists and evangelical Christians. Psychiatrists and evangelical Christians have now become superficial friends, easily accommodating and frequently relying on one another. Modern psychiatrists have become, for the most part, accepting of but disinterested in the Christian faith, and evangelical Christians are generally accepting of modern psychiatry. Little meaningful dialogue has bridged the mainstream of psychiatry and Christian counseling.

A Christian "pastoral care" movement integrated psychiatric and psychological constructs to some degree in mainline Protestant Christianity, though with occasional caution and unease expressed by theologians, even some who were called liberal. Even here, though, a true debate never emerged. Pastoral counselors were at the forefront among those accepting and implementing the theories of Freud and his successors, especially the theories of Carl Rogers. Rogerian therapy dominated pastoral care through much of recent history.

As psychiatry has deemphasized Freudian and Rogerian therapies, opportunities for conversation between pastoral care and psychiatry have been limited. Pastoral counseling and psychiatry have evolved in parallel with little or no crossfertilization in recent years. Yet an industry of Christian counseling has emerged over the past twenty-five years among evangelical Christians. Though the leaders of this industry initially attacked psychiatry, these attacks faded quickly, and today evangelical Christian counseling works in parallel with both pastoral care and psychiatry, stimulating little conversation or debate.

I cannot deny that my concerns derive in part from my inability to integrate my spiritual and professional lives—that is, at times there appears to be little relationship between the two. Integration is a developmental task to which I have devoted many hours of thought and prayer, a task that will never be completed. My own efforts will be unique to me and scarcely of interest to the reader. What drives me to write this book is the sense of a work that is incomplete for many of the patients with whom I have spent years, frustrating years at times, observing their spiritual adaptation to severe emotional problems. I believe that conversation can develop our understanding of and increase our ability to care for these patients, and therefore it is of great importance to psychiatrists.

Where can I begin? Perhaps this is the least difficult task. I begin with the experiences that led me to become disturbed about my own comfortable life. I present the stories of three persons whom I have treated as a psychiatrist and who have raised questions for me which remain unanswered. I have worked with each of these persons for over ten years. They have suffered emotional problems, lived within influential Christian communities and expressed strong Christian beliefs.[3] As a Christian in a similar faith tradition and as a practicing psychiatrist who has lived and worked with these people, I remain uncertain about my understanding of their problems and my attempts to help them. The descriptions are limited, and the questions I raise are far from comprehensive or focused. Nevertheless, the questions probe soul, the relationship of these persons with God and others, and mind, the understanding of their problems in the context of relationships.

1

Stories & Questions

T*he best doctors are the doctors* who know the stories of their patients as well as their diagnoses. These stories are stories of emotional suffering through time in relation to others and to God. The most secure persons in a faith tradition, such as Christianity, are those who know the stories, not just the doctrines, of their faith and who tell their stories of pain within the tradition of these larger stories. A person's life is an ever-evolving story, a story that may well include an episode of severe emotional pain, or what psychiatrists label a psychiatric disorder. The episode cannot be divorced from the story, however, and good doctoring requires good story listening.

Healing of emotional pain, we know intuitively (even if we never read a sentence from Freud), may result from good storytelling. Yet stories leave many questions unanswered, for stories, especially complex stories of emotional pain, are not easily cataloged and filed away. Stories, by their nature, leave loose ends.

The stories of some patients I have treated, even when the treatment was a "success," have raised questions that lead me to believe something is missing from the conversation between psychiatry and Christianity. So it is that I begin my argument with three stories. The questions raised by the stories are not answered in this chapter but rather used as examples of current interactions between psychiatry and Christianity. I attempt to provide some answers, or at least a direction toward answers, in the last chapter of this book, along with another story of a patient. Both the questions and a step toward answering the questions can best be found in stories.

Barbara and Her Demons

I first met Barbara over fifteen years ago. She asked me to be her psychiatrist because she learned I was a Christian. At the time, most church leaders in the Durham, North Carolina, area knew the psychiatry faculty of Duke University included some evangelical Christians.

From the perspective of modern psychiatry, Barbara's emotional suffering was not difficult to explain. She suffered from schizophrenia, a condition in which persons have difficulty telling the real from the unreal. Schizophrenia is loosely associated with madness or insanity and represents the most severe of the mental illnesses, an illness that virtually everyone attributes to faulty brain functioning. Yet schizophrenia, like all so-called mental illnesses, is not easy to actually understand, as Barbara exemplifies.

Treated by numerous psychiatrists, both in private practice and at mental health centers through much of her adult life, Barbara had taken almost every known psychotropic medication at one time or another. At the age of thirty, when I met her, she was living with her mother. She had worked at numerous jobs, none for very long, but was not currently working. She had applied for social security disability because of the difficulty she encountered in maintaining a job. Each job, after a few days or weeks, became too stressful for her to manage, and she would suddenly resign.

As best I could determine, Barbara was rarely released from a position because she was thought to be a poor worker. Barbara herself was convinced that she was beset by demons, evil beings who were attempting to undermine her faith and cause her to do things she knew to be wrong. At times these demons would speak so loudly and persistently that she could not maintain her concentration. She would sit for hours by herself conversing with them. When the demons came, she could not work.

Barbara's "demons" are typical of the symptoms of schizophrenia. When they afflicted her, she could not tell the real from the unreal. At other times, however, the demons left her alone, and she desired to work and to develop a more active social life.

Barbara's mother worked regularly in a restaurant and barely earned enough money to cover rent and food for Barbara and herself. Barbara's father had died when she was six years old, and she had no siblings. While her mother worked, Barbara was forced to remain at home, because they lived far from public transportation. Because her mother worked as many as eighty hours a week, Barbara had few social interactions, except through the local Baptist church, which they attended regularly on Sundays.

At the time I first met Barbara, she was taking multiple medications, including Mellaril (an antipsychotic drug used frequently to treat schizophrenia), Pamelor (an antidepressant), Artane (a drug to counteract the side effects of Mellaril) and Valium (an antianxiety drug). No medications she had taken, past or present, had effectively quieted her demons. Nevertheless, when Barbara occasionally decided to stop taking her medications, she would almost always end up being admitted to the hospital.

Overall, antipsychotic medications have proved effective in calming the symptoms of schizophrenia. Medications such as Thorazine, Mellaril and Haldol are primarily responsible for the dramatic decrease in the numbers of persons requiring long-term care in psychiatric hospitals (especially large state-supported hospitals). Barbara exhibited an amazing tolerance for the medications, for she could take large doses of many drugs and experience virtually no side effects.

From the onset I enjoyed my sessions with Barbara, for she seemed to be a genuinely caring and warm person. Unlike many persons who are diagnosed with schizophrenia, Barbara was easy for me to feel "in touch" with. She would suggest books I should read (frequently evangelical writings that she had found valuable and interesting) and would call at times to learn how I was doing or to wish me a good day. She told me that she often prayed for me because she knew my job must be a difficult one.

Despite her financial problems, Barbara has almost always found a way to pay her psychiatric bills, and on the rare occasions when she could not pay my fees immediately, she apologized profusely. Because of the expense, I suggested to Barbara that she should consider returning to the mental health center, where she could receive her care free of charge. Yet she has insisted that she wished to continue to see me.

Barbara has exhibited some rather bizarre behaviors over the years I have known her. The way she dresses at times is inappropriate and even embarrassing. She might mix pieces of clothing such as blue jeans and a miniskirt, or wear socks that are two different colors. She often does not comb her hair, and she smears lipstick across her face as if she had no mirror. Barbara speaks and laughs so loudly that I often fear our conversations are disturbing my colleagues, even though our offices are relatively soundproof. She frequently laughs for no apparent reason.

The above symptoms easily fit Barbara into the diagnostic category of schizophrenia. To be diagnosed as schizophrenic according to our modern methods for assigning diagnoses, a person must exhibit certain unusual symptoms for many months and experience disability from those symptoms. Barbara experiences delusions, or false beliefs, such as the belief that she is beset by demons. She experiences hallucinations, or false perceptions, such as hearing demons speak to her. She exhibits an inappropriate affect; that is, her emotional responses often don't fit the situation. Her functioning has decreased, for she cannot work, and she has become socially isolated. The deterioration in Barbara's functioning even affects her personal hygiene and grooming.

Yet Barbara is more than a diagnosis of schizophrenia. I have found a person beneath those symptoms, a person who appears to possess a real and persistent faith, a person who is a well-integrated member of an evangelical Christian community.

Neither Barbara nor her mother has developed many social interactions. Having spoken with her mother over the years, I am convinced that she loves Barbara, feels a responsibility for her and tolerates her strange behavior, but has little understanding of the cause of Barbara's problems. Though Barbara's mother does n express strong religious convictions, she and Barbara have found a congregation of Christians in their small town and have become active members. Other members visit Barbara during the week, take her to social gatherings on occasion, and provide her with transportation to and from the church at least two times per week in addition to the Sunday mornings when Barbara and her mother attend together. Before I met Barbara, members of her congregation had attempted to find work for her on a number of occasions. Yet upon recognizing Barbara's inability to work, they have not pressured her to do so. They have not provided financial assistance to Barbara or her mother, but I suspect they would do so if asked. This congregation is known for its care of the disadvantaged and disenfranchised in the community, so Barbara is not alone in being cared for by its members.

Despite the lack of interest in religion among Barbara's family members, the community in which she lives is a very religious community. When Barbara was in elementary school, most of her friends attended church regularly, and Barbara began to attend with them without protest from her parents. She was well integrated into her local church when she first began to experience serious emotional problems.

At sixteen, Barbara was hospitalized for one month at a state mental institution. She had become totally dysfunctional and constantly spoke of demons possessing her. Placed on medications to treat her mental problems, she improved while in the hospital. She did not express as much concern with the demons upon taking the medications. When she was released from the hospital, she was able to return to her school and church. She attended a community mental health center and received medications while simultaneously receiving counseling from her pastor. In addition, some older women in the congregation made themselves available to her, not only to counsel her but to help her with routine daily activities.

The local psychiatrist encouraged Barbara to become active in programs provided by the mental health center. Barbara never participated in those programs, however, and before I began to see her, her sole psychiatric treatment had been medications. The pastor who counseled her had little interest in communicating with the doctors at the mental health center, and despite Barbara's bizarre behavior, he was satisfied with the counsel he provided and the support provided by the congregation.

Barbara expresses appreciation for her Christian friends but rarely speaks of them. It is only upon questioning that I learn how actively and intimately she is involved with the congregation and how frequently they assist her. She acknowledges that she could not function without their help but doesn't dwell on their value to her. Instead Barbara speaks of her beliefs. "I know God has a special mission for me. I think he has called me to be a missionary." Since I have known her, she has sought to find the best way she can serve God. At times she has desired to be a minister, a teacher, even a psychiatrist. She speaks often of projects she has initiated, projects that are never carried to completion. On one occasion she is writing a book; on another, she has begun a course of study toward a divinity school degree by correspondence.

During all the years I have known Barbara, I cannot pinpoint what she actually believes. For example, at times she expresses total confidence that God has saved her from the devil. At other times she is convinced God has punished her with demons and damnation for reasons she cannot know. I am convinced that much of the time (though I don't know how much) the content of her religious thinking is strongly influenced by her schizophrenic disorder. Nevertheless, I do not doubt the reality of Barbara's faith.

Her faith has been the one consistent theme in Barbara's life. I believe that faith and the support she receives from her Christian community have kept her from frequent psychiatric hospitalizations and excessive use of psychiatric services other than medications. The one consistent thread in the story of Barbara's life, a life that to an outsider may appear a fragmented failure, is her belief that she is growing and developing as a Christian. The one aspect of her life that has grown is her faith. She has not been productive in maintaining a job, developing a wider range of social relations or taking on more independent tasks and responsibilities.

Barbara puzzles me. I now see Barbara about once every month for thirty minutes. I check to see that she is taking her medications, for it has become apparent that when she ceases taking medicines the demons return. I encourage her to continue participating in her local congregation, for at times she believes the demons have entered the congregation and she seeks to distance herself. I have encouraged her to return to school, work with the community mental health center through some of their daycare programs, and obtain work in a sheltered workshop, all to no avail.

In the final analysis, Barbara is much as she was when I met her over fifteen years ago. She has not been admitted to the hospital nearly as often, yet I can point to few objective signs of success. Barbara, however, seems most happy and content with my treatment of her. I believe that I have in some way become part of her Christian community—a necessary part, as I am the person who will prescribe the medications she clearly needs. Yet Barbara raises many questions relevant to the conversation between psychiatry and Christianity.

Who is Barbara? I don't believe I can effectively work with Barbara as her psychiatrist unless I know her and she knows me. I also don't believe Barbara's pastor and her closest friends in the congregation can work effectively with Barbara until they know her and she knows them. I suspect that those who relate to Barbara in her congregation are as puzzled as I am as to who she is. In fact, some of them have told me so. They have asked me to "explain" what is going on with her.

One barrier I encounter in coming to know Barbara is that she is easily labeled. By any psychiatrist's description, Barbara is "schizophrenic." By any religious description, Barbara is a Baptist. Though the expression of her religious faith is at times bizarre, few question that Barbara can be classified as an evangelical Christian of the Baptist variety. She calls herself a Baptist, and her church accepts her as a Baptist. By her functional capacity, both federal and local governments label Barbara "disabled." She receives social security benefits and has rarely been questioned as to whether she qualifies for them. A casual encounter with Barbara would lead most of us to simply label her as "crazy" or perhaps "strange."

So Barbara is a crazy Baptist, a disabled schizophrenic. Each of these labels places a barrier to relationships between Barbara and those around her. When we fit her into the Procrustean bed of schizophrenia and disabled, a treatment is perhaps easier to prescribe. Labeling her a schizophrenic renders the prescription of an antipsychotic drug, such as Mellaril, easy. Labeling her Baptist enables her congregation to meet specific needs that she presents to them, for they feel responsible for her. Yet these labels constrain both me as her psychiatrist and her Christian community.

Barbara can be humorous on occasion, and I genuinely laugh with her, not at her. She frequently calls to inquire how I am doing and seems to recognize stresses I feel, stresses that few others recognize. At times Barbara decides that she needs to improve her life with the help of God, such as losing weight, and then she proceeds to lose forty pounds—a demonstration of will not often observed in schizophrenia. Therefore Barbara transcends the labels attached to her. There is a person in there, but we have placed a barrier between that person and ourselves.

Books have been written on personhood, and I have no desire to define this intuitive concept.[1] Suffice it to say that some*body,* not some*thing,* confronts me when I encounter Barbara. A conversation between psychiatry and Christianity, a conversation between Barbara's pastor and me, may help us to know Barbara, to know the person, not just the label.

What can Barbara do? What should she do? Barbara is a person embedded in a culture, a community. That culture and community, however, have unclear expectations for Barbara. On the one hand, she should be able to work. Her bizarre thinking should not control her behavior. She should socialize; she should gradually attain independence from her mother, given that her mother will almost surely die before Barbara and there will be no one to care for her. Yet society is not certain what Barbara is capable of doing or whether its expectations for her are appropriate. She receives mixed messages, for the government has willingly provided her with an income through social security, and her congregation has accepted her dependency and even her bizarre behavior with few questions.

I have encouraged Barbara to seek employment, return to school and seek living arrangements away from her mother. She has been, for the most part, unwilling or unable to follow through with any of these suggestions. At times her Christian community has attempted to discipline her because she has expressed beliefs they find strange, even heretical. They have been quick to criticize some behaviors, such as her unwillingness to give up smoking. Nevertheless, they have placed little pressure on her to become less dependent on the congregation.

I'm not certain if Barbara has goals for the future or is capable of setting long-range goals. She expresses wishes regarding the future, most of which, in my view, are unrealistic. These goals change almost monthly. At least fifty times during the last fifteen years I have heard her express an earnest desire to return to work, but she has not returned to work. I do hear an occasional regret from Barbara—that is, she desires to be productive and have a normal life like people around her. At times she regrets not having children. At other times, however, she seems perfectly content with herself and thanks God that he has blessed her as much as he has. God's blessings, according to Barbara, are the health of her mother, a visit from a friend or a book she has enjoyed reading.

In late-twentieth-century America, the health care industry has little patience with psychiatrists who have been as objectively unsuccessful as I have in improving Barbara's functioning. Soon, I anticipate, I will be encouraged to see Barbara less frequently and to develop a more comprehensive treatment plan with clear goals that demonstrate the effectiveness of the medication I am prescribing and include a more comprehensive, behaviorally oriented and structured plan of care, with the ultimate goal of returning Barbara to the workplace. I can claim that I have reduced the time Barbara would have spent in the hospital over the fifteen years I have treated her, but I can't claim much more.

It is possible, too, that Barbara's Christian community will change its orientation toward her. Situated in a small North Carolina town and characterized by mutual assistance much more than self-sufficiency, this Christian community is unusual. A new pastor with a different orientation, conflict leading to tension within the congregation, or countless other problems may arise to change this congregation and bring it in concert with the American religion of individuality, self-sufficiency and personal responsibility. Members of the congregation may lose patience with Barbara's dependency and her frequent yet unrealized plans to get a job, return to school or perform countless other tasks.

I worry about Barbara if these changes occur. I suspect she cannot (or will not) return to work. If the delicate balance that has been established between her psychiatric care and the support she receives from her faith community is disrupted, the consequences for Barbara, I believe, will be tragic.

Yet I have no way of knowing if I am correct in my belief. Perhaps I have been too patient with Barbara. Perhaps I see more in her perceived comfortable (for the most part) relationship with God than is actually there and less potential for independent living than is there. Perhaps the congregation she takes part in is a fantasy, an unrealistic and sheltered environment that has controlled her and limited her ability to develop.

A conversation between psychiatry and Christianity could provide some answers to these questions. After fifteen years, I have few answers and her congregation has few answers. Barbara, her psychiatrist and her faith community continue to muddle through.

Jason's Unusual Pain

Jason was thirty years old when I first met him eleven years ago. Like Barbara, he came to me because I was known as a Christian psychiatrist. He was not at all convinced, however, that his problem was psychiatric. In fact, he did not believe in mental illness, arguing instead that what is labeled as mental illness in our society is actually sin. If a person lived her or his life as God commanded, then that person would be free of emotional pain, or at least would demonstrate the willpower to live a productive Christian life in the midst of pain.

Jason was no idealist, however. He did not expect to be joyful on all occasions. Life had been a struggle for him, and he had become discouraged at many times during his adolescence and young adult years.

Jason described himself as having been a fairly normal teenager. Though he rarely got in trouble, he did not view himself as particularly moral. He attended a mainline Protestant church on a semiregular basis yet was not raised in a religious family. He felt very little pressure or expectation from his family about his beliefs and behavior. He did not apply himself "as well as I could have" during his studies in high school but graduated with grades sufficient to enter a community college. He later transferred to a state university and finished with a degree in business. He then managed a fast-food restaurant in a small community while taking additional courses in accounting at a nearby college. Upon completing these courses, he moved into our area and found work as the controller for a medium-sized business.

Jason married an elementary school teacher about six months after completing his degree.

Jason's religious experiences set him apart from his peers. In college, he admitted, he was "drifting" and periodically would lose focus, neglect his studies and sit for hours wondering, *What's the meaning of all of this?* As a sophomore, he was asked to attend a Bible study. Impressed by the enthusiasm, focus and guidance of the Bible study leader, he became a regular attendee. The study was sponsored by a local church that had gained a reputation for being very aggressive in evangelism and, to some degree, cultlike. Jason was aware of the reputation of this church but had "not thought much about it." A couple of weeks after joining the Bible study, Jason began to attend the church. Subsequently he became more and more involved in the social life of this religious group. He met his future wife soon after joining the church, where she was also a member.

Jason believed his life dramatically changed once he was "saved" within this church. There was no turning back. He had to commit himself totally to a life of service for Jesus Christ. Yet he described himself as an "infant," in need of much guidance. A single man, approximately Jason's age, became his spiritual mentor. He advised Jason about virtually every aspect of his life, from study habits to gaining experience in personal evangelism. Not only did Jason attend Bible studies, he would invite acquaintances and even strangers to the studies. After approximately two years, he began to study the Bible independently with these persons, serving in turn as their spiritual mentor. He believes at least twelve persons became members of the church directly because of his influence.

Jason did not appear to suffer from his extreme religious devotion. His grades improved, though never exceeding the average for the school. He spent time with his parents, and though his attempts to convert them to his newfound faith were ineffective, their relationship did not deteriorate. They did not express particular concern with Jason's religious beliefs. Jason's wife, Mary, shared a similar devotion to the work of the church, around which their lives were centered. When he was forced to move to find work, Jason and his wife purposely selected our area because there he found a similar religious group.

The moodiness, lack of direction and lack of focus that Jason described as typical of him when he was a high-school student and during his first year of college had virtually disappeared when he joined this religious group. His energy level had never been so high, his mood was constantly up (though not bubbling over), and he genuinely enjoyed both the people in his congregation and the people with whom he worked. At times he would run into difficulties because of his excessive evangelistic efforts at work, but in general he appears to have been well accepted on the job. In my interactions with Jason, his extreme devotion was always evident. Nevertheless, he was easy to talk with, and I found him extremely pleasant.

Jason described his unusual pain as follows. He had recently been passed over for a work promotion that he believed he deserved. Though he realized that "this is not the most important thing in my life," he was extremely disappointed. One night he awakened and felt a sharp, severe pain that seemed to have "virtually cut me in half." He remembers wanting to cry but could not explain the source of the tears. In retrospect, his mood had been less "joyful" prior to this experience of pain; he had experienced difficulty concentrating at work, and his energy had decreased. Nevertheless, he continued to perform his work without major problems and continued his religious practices as before. He was concerned, however, that his "prayer life" was not what it should be. Specifically, he complained that though he would spend forty-five minutes to an hour every morning (a practice he'd begun in college) in prayer and devotion, he had difficulty concentrating during his prayers and wondered whether he was communicating effectively with God. He discussed his problematic prayer life with his spiritual mentor and was encouraged to search for any sins that may have crept into his life and placed a barrier between him and God. Jason, however, could not identify anything that was especially "sinful." His mentor, after consulting the pastor, decided that Jason should be referred for a psychiatric evaluation.

I had little difficulty labeling Jason's psychiatric problem. He was experiencing an episode of depression, what psychiatrists call major depression with melancholia. His mood had changed, and he had clearly lost interest in activities that once were either pleasant or stimulating. This mood change was clear and persistent despite the fact that Jason had, for all practical purposes, not changed his everyday behavior. I dated the onset to about two months prior to the time I first saw him. Previously devoted to exercise, he had ceased exercising and subsequently gained about five pounds. Weight gain was unusual for Jason. He experienced difficulty sleeping. Though he fell asleep as soon as he turned off the lights, he usually would awaken at two or three o'clock in the morning without being able to return to sleep. He used this time in prayer but did not feel the prayer was "getting through" to God.

Jason constantly felt tired, and his wife recognized that his interests, especially his interest in sex, had decreased significantly. He had been told when he joined his church that a husband was responsible for initiating sexual intercourse three times a week, and he made every effort to continue his responsibility to his wife. Mary, however, had become frustrated because intercourse now seemed a chore to him rather than a pleasure. Jason made some mistakes at work—mistakes that he caught easily enough, yet mistakes that in the past he would not have made.

When I suggested to Jason that he was suffering from a "biological depression, a chemical imbalance," he could not comprehend my explanation. He did not "feel" depressed and was as hopeful about the future when I first met him as he had been in the past. If he could only get his life right with God, he would be OK. Yet Jason knew something else was wrong. He focused on the unusual pain. Something must have gone wrong with his brain. He feared that he had suffered something like a stroke or another neurological abnormality. He did not attribute this problem to any supernatural force such as the devil, yet he was frustrated that his faith did not assist him in overcoming the pain.

Jason was impatient for the problem to improve so that he could return to his usual activities at church as well as at work. The members of his church expressed an equal impatience. Two months was just too long to let something "get you down." Though initially supportive, his mentors began to question the sincerity of Jason's faith, as he repeatedly complained that the problem had not improved. They also expressed extreme ambivalence about his seeking psychiatric consultation, even from a Christian psychiatrist. They knew that I did not condone many of their cultlike practices, especially the excessive control the leaders of the church exerted over their members. On the other hand, they found themselves facing a problem that they had difficulty explaining and correcting. They had no desire to lose Jason from their congregation. He had been a productive member for over three years locally, as well as the seven years he had been a member in the city where he attended college.

The religious group to which Jason belonged was a splinter group from a large evangelical denomination. This splinter group was especially reactive to the lack of spirituality and spiritual discipline within the mainline church. The leaders were predominantly under thirty, tended to be dynamic and upbeat, and had been successful in many cities throughout the United States "planting and growing congregations." The local congregation had grown from a core group of fewer than 35 persons to over 250 in five years. Jason and his wife had moved to our area in part to assist in the evangelistic efforts of this young congregation and had been effective in doing just that. The group was noted for its denial of any tradition (secular or sacred) and avoided any authority outside its own boundaries. For example, formal religious training was frowned upon, formal counseling training was thought to undermine the discipline and unity of the church, and formal psychiatric therapy was questioned (but on this the church had not established a clear position). The church had no hesitation to refer persons to physicians for physical illness. They did not believed in faith healing, though they did pray for the sick. I suspect their interpretation of Jason's problem fell somewhere between their recognition that some biological problems disturb the brain and their suspicion of the value of secular psychiatry compared to the counsel of the church leaders.

I told Jason he should take an antidepressant medication. Specifically, I recommended the medication imipramine. Imipramine is a standard medication prescribed to persons suffering from severe depressive episodes. Like most antidepressants, the drug is not an "upper" and is not addictive; it is effective in treating the more severe episodes of depression.

I also told Jason that I would like to see him on a semiregular basis so we could discuss his problems in more detail, and he was willing to do this provided that his spiritual mentors agreed. He reported later that his mentors readily accepted his use of medication. As long as I did not see Jason too frequently, they also accepted my psychotherapy. I believe, however, if I had suggested a more frequent, intense or probing psychotherapy, his Christian community would have responded negatively to my treatment and encouraged Jason to seek care elsewhere, perhaps from a primary care physician who would have only prescribed the medication. Jason would have taken the advice of the leaders of his congregation and ceased working with me.

Jason responded well to imipramine. His sleep improved almost immediately, and after three weeks his energy increased, his concentration improved, and he exhibited more interest in sex as well as other activities that had been of interest to him in the past. If I had simply rated Jason on a scale of symptom improvement, he was a "cure," for his scores on traditional symptom scales went from the moderately severe range to the normal range over the first four weeks that he took imipramine.

In reasonably good conscience, I could have dismissed Jason and followed him for periodic but infrequent checks regarding the use of his medication until the drug was no longer needed. From the perspective of his Christian community, Jason's therapy was also a success. His complaints to the community decreased, and he became as effective and energetic as he had been prior to the depressive episode.

Nevertheless, I remained troubled by one aspect of Jason's recovery, namely, his own perception of what had happened. Jason never integrated his experience with depression into his life story. The event puzzled and troubled him, and he continued to search for an explanation. I saw Jason about once a month during the first six months of his treatment, each time for an hour. During this hour I spent much time (perhaps too much time) explaining to Jason that he suffered a biological illness, a major depression with melancholia, which had responded well to medications. Though Jason felt that something had happened to his brain, he could not accept that his feelings derived from a chemical imbalance and his pain could respond to a medication. He initially wished to stop the medication as soon as possible to demonstrate that he had control over his depressive symptoms. He did try, on two occasions unknown to me during the first six months, to decrease the dose. Each time he reduced the dose, the depressive symptoms recurred: he could not sleep, and the pain returned. After six months Jason accepted the medication, for he recognized that he functioned better when took it, but he was not pleased that he was dependent on it. A responsible individual, a person with a will who could either accept or reject "the ways of the Lord," should not be captive to a medication, especially a medication that influenced the degree to which he could assert his will and experience his relationship with Jesus.

Jason also had difficulty with the prospect that he could not explain, within the context of his life history, why he had experienced such pain and anguish. Why had he become depressed? What had he done? Was God testing him? He was especially troubled because during his experience with depression he doubted that God was listening to his prayers. Perhaps God was treating him as he had treated Job.

After Jason experimented and learned that he needed to take the medication in order to prevent a recurrence of depression, he has remained on the medication for the ten years I have worked with him. Every year I attempt to reduce the medication, only to find that he does need to take it to prevent a recurrence. I now see Jason every six months. At the age of forty, Jason has two children and has advanced in his career as an accountant. Seven years after his depressive experience he went through a crisis of faith, as he describes it, and began to question some of the excessive practices of the religious group to which he belonged. His wife had already begun to express doubts about the group. After a period of time during which he and his wife attended no congregation, they began visiting a more traditional evangelical church, where they now are active and content members.

Even today, however, Jason has not integrated the depressive illness into his life story. He has experienced no episodes of severe depression since the initial episode, and the return of symptoms when he has attempted to withdraw the medication has quickly reversed when he has increased the dose. Jason has read widely to try to understand his experience. He has read secular explanations of major depression, evangelical writings on depression and numerous self-help books (both Christian and secular). None have satisfied him. Specifically, Jason cannot accept his need for a medication to offset a chemical imbalance in his brain which had, when those chemicals were "out of balance," led him to feel certain feelings and think certain thoughts. Those thoughts and feelings were alien, they were isolated, they did not fit his perception of himself.

I have assisted Jason as best I can. I am convinced that I could fit such an experience into my own story. I could explain it intellectually, and it would not undermine my faith or my identity. To some extent, my views leave Jason confused and leave me with a sense that I have, even over these many years, never been able to truly empathize with this young man with whom I share many beliefs and much cultural background.

How do persons assimilate a "drug cure" into their sacred journey, their pilgrim's progress, through life? Psychiatrists who examine a person such as Jason have little difficulty interpreting either his emotional pain or his response to the antidepressant drug imipramine. We have little difficulty understanding why Jason must continue on the medication. Some persons are prone to relapse into depression once they have suffered a depressive episode, and extended therapy with an antidepressant drug can prevent such relapses. We can easily dismiss the idea that Jason is "addicted" to imipramine, that imipramine is a crutch he relies on unnecessarily in order to live a relatively normal life. Rather, we view Jason's need of the drug imipramine as similar to the need of a person experiencing congestive heart failure who responds to digitalis. That person is not addicted to digitalis, yet she may take the drug throughout the remainder of her life, for it clearly improves her functioning. The analogy between digitalis and imipramine, to me, is obvious.

This analogy, however, is not obvious to Jason. Despite the descriptions of his depressive episode Jason has given me over the years, and despite his attempt to understand it, to this day I do not understand what Jason experienced. The most parsimonious explanation as to why the episode occurred when it occurred is that it happened spontaneously and was biologically driven. I continue to search with Jason, however, for events in his life that may have contributed to the onset of the depression. To Jason, his depression experience cannot be divorced from his life with others and with God. Despite the disappointment at not being promoted at work, despite the conflicts he encountered along his spiritual journey, Jason has difficulty, and so do I, in pinpointing any events and disruption of relationships that may have precipitated his severe depression.

Jason's depression does not fit his life story because it is "off time"—that is, it did not occur at a time when he would have expected it to occur. Jason would have, perhaps, better accepted his depressive experience if it had occurred prior to his rather dramatic religious conversion, because he was without God and depression could be perceived as the absence of a relationship with God. Even if he had taken a medication and continued to take it for the depression, the fact that he changed his life and his "attitude" following that conversion could enable Jason to understand his depression better. Perhaps if the depression had occurred prior to his leaving the cultlike religious community, he could have associated it with that restrictive environment and then could have associated relief with movement to a more traditional community (and perhaps attributed his recovery to his spiritual growth and development).

Yet he could not correlate the depression with events in his life. Even if Jason could have associated the depression with one of the usual stresses of life, such as loss of a loved one, he could use the depressive episode, his recovery from it and his subsequent growth in faith within a stress/adaptation paradigm. For example, Jason could have viewed the depression episode as a response to a stressor such as the breakup of a romantic relationship which called upon untapped resources within him, resources now available to him because he learned to adapt to failed relationships. Jason has yet to identify any explanation, though, and therefore any value or meaning from the experience of this severe depression.

I don't have a clear answer as to how Jason could integrate this depressive episode into his life story. Perhaps I have overmedicalized his emotional suffering. I doubt, however, that extensive traditional counseling, either with me or with a pastor, would have been of value in facilitating this integration. Jason was not motivated to spend hours with someone else in order to answer this question, for his experience with both religious and secular counseling as well as reading books on depression had been discouraging. He ultimately must find his own answer. For my part, I must find a means of communicating with

Jason, based on psychiatry and theology, that reaches him better than my current communication.

William Styron, in *Darkness Visible,*[2] provides a graphic description of a depressive episode he experienced late in life. Because of Styron's fame and his willingness to expose himself to his readers, and especially to expose the pain of his depression, he has become a popular speaker to psychiatrists and psychiatric patients. My reading of *Darkness Visible* is that Styron struggled to explain his severe depression and was most frustrated with the mental health professionals with whom he worked because they communicated poorly and provided little assistance in helping him understand his depression, as well as failing to treat his depression successfully. For years Styron had written novels that explored characters' desire to explain their external actions based on their innermost feelings. His *The Confessions of Nat Turner* is the prototypical example of such an exploration, even though Styron's interpretation of Turner's behavior in leading a rebellion of slaves against a white community in southeastern Virginia has not been accepted by many African-American activists.[3] From my perspective, the point is that Styron, by nature, searches for meaning, for answers. When he faced his own "darkness," his own journey into depression, he could not accept a medical explanation as the sole explanation. His depressive experience must have been, in his view, related to his life story, especially his relations with others as a child.

Styron caught the attention of psychiatrists not just because he was a well-known writer but because he was struggling with a question that psychiatrists have not been able to help their patients answer: "What is happening to me and why?" Psychiatrists have welcomed the dialogue with Styron, for he not only brought the realities of mental suffering to the attention of the public but also stimulated psychiatrists to reexamine the relationship aspects of their therapies.

Psychiatrists and Christian theologians would have paid much less attention to a book written by Jason. Yet Jason, like Styron, describes a concrete example of an important issue worthy of conversation between psychiatry and Christian theology. How can one fit a severe depressive episode into one's life story, a story of evolving relations with God and one's faith community?

To what extent should a psychiatrist interpret or interfere with religious practices which appear restrictive, even cultist, when those practices do not directly impact the illness of a patient?

I have little doubt that Freud, if he had worked with Jason, would have explored Jason's religious beliefs and practices in depth in the midst of his depression. What personality characteristics and past developmental experiences had contributed to Jason's attraction to the extremely structured and rigid religious group to which he joined himself? What steps in Jason's psychological development would eventually free him from this restrictive group?

When I first met Jason, I had significant concerns about the religious group to which he belonged. I suspected the day would come when Jason would leave the group. Perhaps he would abandon his faith altogether in reaction to the restriction he had experienced for many years. Perhaps he would gravitate to a more traditional, less restrictive group. Yet at the time I first met Jason, it was clear that his restrictive religious environment had not directly contributed to the depression he experienced. He recovered from the depressive episode and his functioning returned to normal through no change in his religious practices nor in the persons with whom he associated.

So I took a focused, empirical approach to the emotional pain experienced by Jason and had little difficulty justifying a hands-off approach toward his religious practices and his faith community. This approach is consistent with modern neuropsychiatry. Interestingly, the restrictive religious community to which Jason belonged also took an empirical, hands-off approach to the treatment of his emotional suffering. The experience Jason reported was alien enough that they did not pursue in depth an explanation of his pain based on his sin or the forgiveness of that sin and subsequent healing within the community. Once Jason recovered from the depression, he returned to the activities in which he had been engaged previously, and to my knowledge no church member probed him about his experience with depression.

The church and I thus achieved an easy accommodation regarding the care of Jason. In practice this accommodation worked well, for Jason received the professional care he required without interference from his religious community, and he was able to work through his relationship with the community without interference from me.

Yet this easy accommodation left me uneasy. To understand Jason as a person necessitates an understanding of the social environment in which he lived and his religious beliefs. For Jason, his "life" was his life in that Christian community. That community influenced, if not controlled, both his beliefs and his social activities. The authority of the community was so great when I first met him that if I had not been given its permission to work with Jason, he would not have sought my help. Surely there are many others within this community who suffer emotional problems and who could potentially benefit from psychiatric care. The community may not be as quick to identify and refer those persons as they were to refer Jason. If I am to be concerned as a mental health professional with the emotional well-being of persons in society as a whole, then I must be concerned about the individual communities in which my patients live. And if the leaders of Jason's religious community are to responsibly discharge their duties to relieve the emotional suffering of their members, they should learn to work effectively with psychiatry. Their community is a magnet for persons with severe psychiatric problems, given their aggressive evangelistic approach. They promise friendship, guidance and support to persons struggling to survive the stress of modern life. They reach out to help those who are seeking help.

Psychiatrists dismissing this cultic community out of hand would, I fear, place a barrier in front of many persons who could benefit from psychiatric care. For the cultic community to dismiss psychiatry out of hand would erect a similar barrier. Yet productive conversation between this community of Christians and psychiatrists will be difficult at best.

Betty, the Amateur Psychiatrist

Betty first sought my care fifteen years ago for severe panic attacks. Through her own reading, she had recognized her problem as a disorder that potentially could be treated through psychiatric therapy. As with Jason, Betty's problem was relatively easy to identify, and her treatment was successful.

Though she sought my assistance initially because I was a "Christian psychiatrist," I heard little about her faith or her Christian community during the first two or three months of therapy. Betty was a member of a large evangelical Protestant church. She viewed her faith as secure and her problem circumscribed enough that a long, detailed exploration of her beliefs and how they might be contributing to her problem or its solution appeared superfluous from the outset to her, and I did not pursue her beliefs aggressively.

Betty's problem was that she would experience periods of intense fear or discomfort, usually lasting only a couple of minutes, yet paralyzing her when they occurred. These attacks occurred approximately two times per week and had increased in frequency before I began seeing her. Though she remembered infrequent attacks (once every six months or once every year) since she was an adolescent, the problem had become more disabling when she reached the age of thirty, the age at which I first saw her. These attacks were characterized by a sense of smothering, lightheadedness, palpitations, an accelerated heart rate, numbness in her extremities, chest pain and a sense that she was about to die. The attacks would spontaneously occur and disappear. Though they did not awaken her at night, they might occur at any other time during the day, and she had been forced to limit many of her activities, especially driving. Between these episodes of panic she felt a mild but persistent anxiety, an anxiety no worse than what she had experienced since adolescence and that did not interfere with her usual activities.

Betty responded well to therapy. I explained the nature of panic attacks to her, an explanation she readily accepted. I told her that some persons are prone to develop episodes of extreme anxiety, which are in part biological in origin and can be virtually disabling if they occur frequently. These episodes, however, can be controlled with treatment. We would work together using two approaches to therapy, one pharmacological and one behavioral. She began taking imipramine at night. Imipramine, the antidepressant taken by Jason, has also been demonstrated to be effective in preventing panic episodes. I told her that we could prescribe an antianxiety agent, such as Xanax, but we should first determine whether the imipramine was effective. I also instructed Betty in some techniques for relaxation and suggested that she practice these techniques two or three times a day. She was an apt learner and was persistent in practicing the relaxation along with imagery of a peaceful scene. For Betty, that peaceful scene was a pasture surrounded by trees and traversed by a babbling brook. She imagined that she reclined in the pasture, heard the brook in the background, watched the clouds slowly moving overhead and felt at one with God and his creation.

Betty responded well to imipramine and relaxation therapy. Within one month the panic attacks virtually disappeared, and she described her overall level of anxiety as having declined significantly. She experienced few side effects from the medication and was willing to continue taking it as long as necessary. We agreed, since the therapy had been effective, that I would see her infrequently, primarily to adjust the dose of medication and to make certain that she was not experiencing side effects.

For fifteen years Betty has taken imipramine. On a number of occasions we tried, unsuccessfully, to withdraw the drug. Each time she experienced a return of panic episodes. Except in those periods when she was off medications, the panic episodes have been infrequent, usually occurring two or three times a year. Otherwise Betty has experienced virtually no problems and has been functioning normally.

If this were the end of the story, there would not appear to be any necessity for conversation between psychiatry and Christianity regarding Betty. She sought psychiatric help, was treated, improved and returned to her usual activities with no concern expressed by her pastor, fellow church members or herself about conflicts with her faith. In contrast to Jason, she views her illness as primarily biological, an illness that can be controlled by routine psychiatric therapies, and has had no difficulties integrating the illness into her overall life story. The problem that arose with Betty was unexpected: she became infatuated with the effectiveness of psychiatric therapy.

Prior to the period of frequent panic attacks, Betty had been neither opposed to nor strongly supportive of psychiatry. She had friends, both within her Christian community and without, who had suffered psychiatric illnesses, and she had been supportive of them without expressing much interest in their psychiatric therapy. In fact, Betty interacted with many individuals suffering emotional pain. Betty was a helper. Perhaps bordering on being a "busybody," Betty had an uncanny ability to recognize people, especially in her church, who were suffering emotional problems. She sought them out, took them to breakfast or lunch, encouraged them to tell her about their problems, prayed with them, assisted them in whatever way she could and rallied other persons in her congregation to do the same. Betty was the hub of a network within her congregation that supported persons experiencing emotional pain, and this network was most effective. Her pastor and other church leaders recognized the effectiveness of this network and frequently called on Betty, as an informal coordinator, to identify individuals who could provide various kinds of assistance for needy people, from counseling regarding marital problems to simple help with everyday tasks of living. Having never been in need of a helping relationship herself prior to experiencing the panic disorder, Betty had thought little of the professional services that might be needed to heal the emotions. She believed in informal helping relations.

All this changed once Betty responded to medication and instruction in relaxation. She became my biggest fan and began to refer to me virtually everyone she knew with emotional problems. I could not see all of them, so I referred most of them to other colleagues. In some cases the referrals were appropriate, and the individuals responded to psychiatric care and returned to their families and communities more productive. In other cases, however, the individuals either entered into long and nonproductive relationships with psychiatrists or quickly backed away from psychiatric care. But this mixed success rate did not deter Betty. Psychiatry was the answer!

Betty became extremely active in a support group made up of people suffering from panic disorder. Within a couple of years she was the leader of this group and had recruited many persons to it. She became personally acquainted with over ten local psychiatrists known for their interest in and expertise with panic disorder. Betty also accumulated a library of self-help books and books explaining panic disorder and other psychiatric problems. Each time I saw her, she asked if I was aware of a good book on some psychiatric topic. Often she found self-help books herself when visiting bookstores and brought me copies. None of these books had a Christian perspective. They usually were written by mental health professionals to explain mental illnesses to laypersons. I have used with benefit many of the books Betty identified for me. Most are easily read and accurately describe common psychiatric disorders, such as depression, panic disorder and obsessive-compulsive disorders.

Betty continues as a member of her congregation. Yet the network of women and men that she was instrumental in establishing and maintaining faded to the background of her interests. Betty now seeks volunteers for and applies her organizational skills to secular self-help groups for mental disorders. She communicates only infrequently with her pastor regarding the needs of her church. Instead she casts her net much wider to search for persons needing assistance. She continues to arrange appointments with psychiatrists and psychologists for these contacts so that their problems may be treated. Betty has found her mission in life, or at least has found a new one. She expends as much, if not more, energy as a spokesperson for psychiatry as she originally expended in facilitating a healing community within her congregation.

I cannot imagine a better friend of psychiatry than Betty, but I perceive that she is now peripheral to her Christian community as opposed to an integral part. From what Betty tells me, few if any of her Christian friends "understand" mental illness and the need for professional help, and she therefore looks upon them as uneducated. She does spend time attempting to instruct them about the marvels of modern psychiatry but believes that her efforts have been less successful in her church than among her neighbors, and especially among the mental health support groups with which she has worked.

Should I, as a psychiatrist, encourage Betty to become more realistic about the limitations of psychiatry? Psychiatry, as a specialty of medicine, has since its inception sought respect from society. Respect, at least among the educated, peaked during the years when psychoanalysis dominated psychiatry. Today, however, psychiatry suffers a lack of respect even though psychiatrists are now more capable of relieving emotional suffering than ever before. We need all the support we can garner. People such as Betty are among our most valued friends. They dispel the myth that psychiatrists are ineffective and patients with psychiatric illnesses are hopeless and carry a stigma.

Betty is a personable, outgoing, "together" kind of person. Though she is active and at times can be rather aggressive, she is skilled in her interactions with others. Few would question Betty's sanity, and most envy her upbeat attitude, her knowledge and her ability to organize and mobilize people. When Betty says psychiatry has something to offer, people listen. Even though I believe Betty has an exaggerated view of the potential of psychiatry, my colleagues and I would think twice about tempering Betty in her quest to improve the status and delivery of mental health services. We need a good relationship with Betty!

When I consider the situation as a Christian, however, Betty presents me with a dilemma. I believe she has made a religion out of psychiatry, has overdetermined the effectiveness of the psychiatrist in the overall care of persons suffering emotionally, and has unwittingly undermined an equally important component of care for emotional suffering—a supportive religious community. Though Betty moved with ease from the Christian community to secular self-help groups, many Christians do not move so easily from religious to secular-based self-help groups. As best I can determine, Betty had been a prime mover in creating a very effective group of women and men providing helping relationships within her congregation. Later, after becoming impressed by her rapid response to treatment of panic disorder, she failed to recognize the good work in which she had been involved in her faith community.

Did Betty respond too easily? Though Betty was not depressed and she did not take Prozac, I believe she falls within a category of individuals who have been "wowed" by their dramatic and beneficial response to psychopharmacological drugs. Don't misunderstand me. Betty was suffering from a psychiatric disorder, and her response was a relief of suffering from that illness, not an artificial "high." Yet she is similar to persons who have become enamored with the wonders of psychopharmacology, the "Prozac Proselytizers" described by Peter Kramer in his book *Listening to Prozac*.[4] Though even Kramer is uncomfortable with the missionary zeal of some persons who advocate psychopharmacology, dramatic cures such as that experienced by Betty are the most positive publicity for psychiatry since the popularity of Freud during the early twentieth century.

Betty has now joined the ranks of those seeking a wonder drug. Melvin Konner, in a recent article in *The New York Times Magazine,* notes that doctors are giving antidepressants to patients who are not mentally ill and that patients like the effects. He asks, "Why not?"[5] Konner describes his own experience with a lifelong depression and how, after years of psychotherapy, he felt "enormously better" after taking a traditional antidepressant, desipramine. In fact, Konner suspects that medications he took later changed his temperament as well as relieved his psychiatric disorder. "For me, the medication became a platform on which I could function in a very different way." The change occurred when he began to take Zoloft (a sibling of Prozac). "Critics would have us to believe that it is good for us to feel the pain, the existential dread, to work through it with friends or therapists or pastors. I tried, for too many years. . . . Critics caution that if we blunt the pain we may fail to deal with the internal and external problems that are causing it. This is a noble sentiment. But why limit it to depression or obsession?" Konner then suggests that taking any medication, such as an analgesic for arthritis, is avoiding pain and therefore perhaps avoiding the realities of life.

Konner makes an important point, and I doubt any rational person would suggest we cease using medications that ease pain and relieve suffering. We must recognize that medications to ease pain date to antiquity; even the prophet Jeremiah asked, "Is there no balm in Gilead?" (Jer 8:22). Nevertheless, I think Konner misses another dimension of emotional suffering, and this dimension is well illustrated by Betty. Konner forgets that *suffering has, for thousands of years, bound people together.* Through most of human history, suffering has been a concern much more of the community than of professionals. Physicians have now entered an era when they have found rather extraordinary means to dramatically relieve some illnesses, including mental illnesses. Yet what happens if we place all of our support and faith in physicians and their new technologies? The community of care is at great risk of dissolving, like the self-help groups so ardently supported by Betty.

For every Betty, for every Melvin Konner, there is someone else who is not nearly so impressed with existing psychiatric therapies. Psychiatry doesn't work for them. Are they to be left to suffer in isolation? Betty had garnered a group of persons in her church to relieve the sense of isolation that naturally accompanies emotional suffering. True, she transferred her interest and support to the community at large, but I wonder why she made the transfer. Perhaps Betty suffers from the same need to specialize that afflicts many of our efforts. Perhaps she needed a specific focus, such as panic disorder, as a platform for providing support. Prior to her treatment for panic disorder, however, she did not need this platform. General support for those experiencing physical and emotional pain within her Christian community was enough.

Considering the Question

The questions I have posed, deriving from the three cases presented above, are not the most profound that could be posed for psychiatrists and Christians. For some readers the answers may appear self-evident, and I may appear naive for not having recognized the obvious answers. Others may critize me for not being content with the successful treatment of Barbara, Jason and Betty.

Yet I ask that you not be too quick to criticize. Each of the persons I have described is someone I know well. I share with them a common faith. I have served as a psychiatrist to each of them for many years, so I have had an interest in their souls—that is, in them as persons in relation to others and to God. I have been cautious in my work with these people in part because they puzzle me, leaving questions unanswered despite superficial success in therapy.

The conversation is ongoing within me. I engage in this conversation at times with my psychiatric colleagues and my Christian brothers and sisters. Yet the hunger for such conversation among my psychiatric and Christian colleagues is meager. I hear some interest, but most of my colleagues are preoccupied with other matters. Nevertheless, I am convinced that the questions I ask probe the heart of the emotional suffering experienced among millions of professing Christians in the Western world today and the issues faced by professionals who treat them.

2

Conversation & Debate

$\mathbf{T}$*he conversation I describe in* chapter one, a conversation that arose in me and has arisen in others, did not emerge from a vacuum. The conversation, the problem, the questions that are unanswered are much like the complaints and problems presented to physicians by their patients.

We designate the concern which opens the dialogue between doctor and patient the "chief complaint." Most chief complaints, however, mean little to the physician until they are placed in their historical context. For example, if a person says, "I am severely anxious, I cannot sit still, I feel as if I am about to jump out of my skin," I immediately begin an inquiry into the context, the history, of that anxiety.

□ "Is this the first time you have been anxious?"

□ "Tell me about yourself."

□ "Tell me about your past."

Only when I understand the context and history of the complaint am I prepared to prescribe a remedy.

The concerns I have about the lack of meaningful conversation between psychiatry and Christianity, my chief complaint, can only be understood in context. Since antiquity, as I describe below, the interrelation between emotional suffering and religion has been a central concern to both philosophers and theologians. Yet in my view only with the writings of Freud did a true conversation and debate arise between psychiatry and Christianity.

Freud brought to the surface the critical need to understand suffering both within the context of psychiatric care and philosophy/theology. This brief historical review is not meant to be complete, and some may view it as biased. Perhaps so, yet the review is history through my eyes, the eyes of a psychiatrist and Christian who is attempting to stimulate an intelligent conversation by presenting my complaint in context. The context is emotional suffering and its treatment in relationship to others and to God.

The Care of Emotional Suffering Before Freud

The world's great religions have reflected upon and struggled with emotional suffering since antiquity.[1] Each has recognized the reality of depression and anxiety as well as provided vehicles for expressing suffering, such as through prayer. King David, in Psalm 31, prayed,

> Be merciful to me, O LORD, for I am in distress;
>> my eyes grow weak with sorrow,
>> my soul and my body with grief.
> My life is consumed by anguish
>> and my years by groaning;
> my strength fails because of my affliction,
>> and my bones grow weak.
> Because of all my enemies,
>> I am the utter contempt of my neighbors; . . .
> For I hear the slander of many;
>> there is terror on every side;
> they conspire against me
>> and plot to take my life. (vv. 9-13)

The inevitability of emotional pain is equally apparent in the Qur'an (2.210):

> Do you reckon that you will enter the garden without there coming upon

you the like of those who have passed before you?

Evils and griefs afflicted them, and they trembled so much that the apostle and those who were with him said, "When will the help of God come?"

Descriptions of emotional suffering have pervaded literature, both sacred and secular, since humankind has recorded its history. Through the centuries of the church, Christians have typically interpreted emotional conflicts as spiritual struggles and expressed little interest in the concept of insanity. Persons since antiquity have through their religions revealed their emotional pain and tried to understand its origins and to gain some relief from their revelations and spiritual explanations. The questions of Jason (see chapter one) are therefore not new.

The apostle Paul, during the first century of the Christian era, was perhaps the earliest Christian writer to express the emotional pain resulting from inner conflict. In Romans 7:7-24 he describes the conflict he felt between the demands of the law and his personal desires:

When I want to do good, evil is right there with me. For in my inner being I delight in God's law; but I see another law at work in the members of my body, waging war against the law of my mind and making me a prisoner of the law of sin at work within my members. What a wretched man I am! Who will rescue me from this body of death? (vv. 21-24)

It is debatable whether the struggle Paul describes is analogous to the struggle between the unconscious and conscience, or superego, drives proposed by Sigmund Freud nearly two thousand years later. Few, however, would debate that Paul experienced a painful emotional struggle and used this struggle as a means to understand the grace of Jesus Christ.

The most profound expression of internal conflict among the early Christians was by Augustine of Hippo (born A.D. 354). After experiencing a conflict of faith which led him to temporarily adopt the aesthetic philosophy of the Manichaeans, he underwent a dramatic conversion to Christianity, which he describes in his *Confessions*. Upon reading a passage of Scripture, he reports,

I cast myself down, I know not how, under a certain fig tree, giving full vent to my tears; and the floods of mine eyes gushed out an acceptable sacrifice to thee. . . . Instantly at the end of this sentence, by a light as it were of serenity infused into my heart, and all the darkness of doubt vanished away.[2]

Augustine has been of interest to modern psychoanalysts because of the introspective method he employed to reach the conclusions upon which he based his faith. That is, Augustine reviewed his life via self-analysis (as did Freud) and revealed in *Confessions* his earliest memories. He also expressed his innermost thoughts without reservation. Augustine told his story, the entire story, and thereby gained relief from his emotional conflict. A psychological interpretation of Augustine's confession might be that introspection lead to understanding himself and thereby he made peace with his past and himself. The interpretation by Augustine was that God made peace with him. Confession wasn't about the business of settling internal conflict; confession was about the soul, that is, his relationship with God.

Robert Burton (1577-1640) reflected copiously upon his mood swings in *The Anatomy of Melancholy.* A humanist thoroughly grounded in the Enlightenment of the seventeenth century, he describes his emotional problems graphically and poetically, though his description is filled with misconceptions about the origins of his melancholy:

When I go musing all alone,
Thinking of divers things fore-known,
When I build castles in the air,
Void of sorry and void of fear,
Pleasing myself with phantasms sweet,
Methinks the time runs very fleet.
All joys to this are folly,
Naught so sweet as melancholy.[3]

To Burton, psychological distress was not only a burden but also a stimulus to gain greater insight into life. He derived knowledge, in part, from confessing his problems to others:

If then our judgment be so depraved, I reasoned over-ruled, well-recip-rocated, then we cannot seek our own good, or moderate ourselves, as in this disease [melancholia] commonly it is, the best way for ease is to impart imagery to some friend, not to smother it up in our own breast;

for grief concealed strangles the soul; but when as we shall but impart to some discreet, trusting, loving friend, it is instantly removed. . . . A friend's counsel is a charm like a Mandrake wine, it allayeth our cares.[4] Novelists of the nineteenth century such as Dostoyevsky, Balzac, Tolstoy and Stendhal continued this soul-searching tradition by emphasizing psychological and spiritual themes, or soul sickness, in their works.[5] In *The Brothers Karamazov* (Dostoyevsky), Ivan wills the death of his obscene and uncaring father. But when he learns his father has been murdered, he is shocked and feels tremendous guilt, though he did not participate in the actual killing. Writing before the time of Freud, Dostoyevsky captures graphically the internal conflict of the introspective son who at once loves and hates his father.[6]

Ivan's psychological conflicts invade his spiritual contemplations as well. He believes in God, yet cannot accept God's world. From this spiritual conflict, Ivan has a vision in which an inquisitor during the Spanish Inquisition places Jesus on trial for his response to the temptations by the devil (Mt 4:1-11): Jesus should have turned the stones of the wilderness into bread, for he could have therefore fed the masses. Jesus should have jumped from the highest point of the temple, for he would have gained the attention of the masses. Jesus should have bowed before the devil, for he would have gained control over the nations in order to perform the greatest good. Ivan's love-hate relationship with his father is projected into a love-hate relationship with Jesus. Dostoyevsky therefore illustrates the conflict which may arise when accepted Christian beliefs are tested by self-analysis of the psyche.

Nineteenth-century philosophers, especially Nietzsche, Schopenhauer and Kierkegaard, also probed the troubled psyche. Kierkegaard resolved his own psychological crisis through conversion to Christianity, though not the traditional faith of his native Lutheran Church. After winning the love of Regina Olson, with whom he was deeply in love, his inner conflicts were so great that he broke off the engagement. This torment marked the beginning of his lifelong work to assist persons in knowing what it truly means to be a Christian.

He believed that God cannot be the object of humankind's thought, but rather the living challenge who forces human beings to make a decision. Persons are not saved by coming to know something; rather, they are saved by the transformation of their existence through divine grace. One can become a Christian only by a leap of faith, a radical commitment of one's life to the divine Other. Though intellectual doubt is never overcome, in a leap of faith humankind can achieve moral certainty.

Nietzsche, in contrast, denied God, the Other, and believed emotional pain can be overcome by recognizing one's own power, the power of the superman. For both Kierkegaard and Nietzsche, however, overcoming emotional suffering begins with confronting a problem with soul, that is, the relationship of the person with others, especially the perceived divine Other.

The Origins of Pastoral Care for Emotional Suffering

Christian clergy have, through history, been among the first to hear of people's emotional problems. Within two hundred years of the death of Jesus, leaders were writing letters and treatises containing instructions about spiritual direction and consolation, repentance and discipline, grief and growth. The clergy viewed their task as the curing of souls and wrote extensively about their various theories for healing the wounded soul. Most of these writings emphasized private guidance and public penance. Following the Protestant Reformation of the sixteenth century, many prescriptive practices of the Catholics were rejected by Protestants. Yet Protestant traditions developed their own practices for healing the emotional wounds.

E. Brooks Holifield describes four patterns for pastoral care of persons with emotional problems which derived from the four major religious traditions in early America.[7] Catholic theologians wrote manual after manual for evoking detailed confessions and prescribing the proper penances. The penitential system reached back for over a thousand years in Catholicism, so Catholics in America continued an age-old process. Emotional suffering could be relieved by reestablishing the relationship of the person with God.

Within the Lutheran tradition, sin was perceived as an incapacity to trust God, exhibited in self-righteousness. Therefore pastoral care consisted not in the enumeration of specific sins but in encouraging feelings of repentance, especially in the community's joint confession at the celebration of the Lord's Supper. Emotional healing came through communion with God and the church.

Anglican ministers practiced pastoral care within the context of an accepted cosmic order. Sin involves a willful breaking of civil peace and religious unity. Pastoral care therefore focused on making certain that all things were done "in a fitting and orderly way" (1 Cor 14:40). The Anglican pastor was involved in every activity of his parish, and pastoral care had to do with maintaining a peaceful and ordered parish. Emotional healing was facilitated by restoring relations within the parish.

Within the Reformed tradition, sin was seen as idolatry. The Puritan pastor therefore became a specialist in the care of the idolatrous heart and looked beneath behavior to motives and feelings. Healing was believed to arise from ensuring a relationship with the true God.

In each of these traditions, the spiritual development of the normal parishioner was the focus of pastoral care. Life is difficult, a "pilgrim's progress" through a world of sin, for every Christian. The pastor emphasized the levels of growth for the Christian through life. For example, the Puritan theologian William Perkins (1558-1602) suggested ten levels of religious growth, beginning with an outward or inward "cross" that exposes the insufficiency of the self. Following a number of works of preparation, grace leads to contemplation, which in turn leads to sparks of faith and finally the joy of heartfelt, voluntary submission to God. The journey of life is a journey toward reconciliation with God and peaceful relationships with others, the necessities of a healthy soul.[8]

The Origins of Medical Treatment of Emotional Suffering

Pastoral care did not include the care of the insane, the severely ill. There is no universal definition of insanity, and some, such as Thomas Szasz, suggest that mental illness is a myth.[9] Yet crosscultural and historical studies verify that some persons in virtually every society are considered to deviate so far from normal behavior that they are labeled "ill" or "insane." They are not treated as persons whose emotional pain can be expected to emerge as a rational response to their circumstance, nor are they held totally responsible for their behavior.[10]

Biological causes for these severe mental problems have been proposed from antiquity. Hippocrates, for example, describes biological causes for hysteria (a wandering uterus) and severe depression (an excess of black bile). Some physicians devoted themselves to the treatment of emotional suffering, so psychiatry as a vocation (though not as a medical specialty) is older than Christianity.

Prior to Freud, however, there was little contact, little conversation, between psychiatry and Christianity. The care of the severely disturbed was not considered a responsibility of the church, either through individual pastoral care or as a social obligation. Humane treatment of severe emotional problems did not emerge until long after the Renaissance of the fifteenth and sixteenth centuries. Even the historical forces that ushered in modern science and spawned humanism had little impact on the treatment of the insane. The mad and the mentally anguished were at times put on ships and entrusted to mariners, for foolishness and water were thought to be made for one another.[11] These "ships of fools" traversed the seas, rivers and canals of Europe with their cargo of the debilitated and the deranged, virtually isolated from society.

Later, the severely mentally ill were isolated in asylums, hidden from society throughout the nineteenth century. Out of sight meant out of mind. The church, which continued to dominate the thoughts and feelings of the common person, expressed little interest in the insane unless they were considered possessed by demons or engaged in pacts with the devil. Some of the women tried and convicted during the 1692 witch hunt in Salem, Massachusetts, would be considered mentally ill today by Christians and non-Christians alike.

The relationship of the severely mentally ill to God and others was not viewed as a special challenge to the church. Rather they were labeled as relating to the devil, at worse, or lacking a relationship with God, at best. For example, the severe depression experienced by persons who had professed a strong faith was termed "religious melancholy." The sixteenth-century physician and clergyman Timothic Bright differentiated between melancholy due to a guilty conscience and "true melancholia."[12]

Along with religious melancholy, the church was forced to confront the passions and catharsis produced by the Great Awakening of the eighteenth century and early nineteenth century. The religious revivals of the Awakening kept pastors busy. The distraught, the anxious and the paranoid came from the cities and the back woods telling their pastors about visions, trances and healings. Those inspired by the Great Awakening included a range of persons, most of whom would not be labeled today as emotionally disturbed, yet scattered among them were persons experiencing severe emotional disturbances. Many, perhaps most, benefited from the revival, yet a few presented a true challenge to the clergy.[13] The problems presented to these pastors precipitated heated debates among the clergy about the human faculties and free will in the process of healing. These encounters did not, however, lead pastors to view severe emotional suffering as innate to humankind. Neither did the debates lead the church to demonstrate concern for persons with the most severe mental problems. Nevertheless, the church clearly was in contact with persons with severe emotional suffering.

Phillippe Pinel, a secular physician, led the crusade for the humane treatment of the mentally ill in Paris during the early nineteenth century. This humane treatment did not result from a concept of soul but rather from biological empiricism.[14] Pinel, from his observation of hospital patients, rejected the view that mental illness results from moral impoverishment or supernatural possession. Instead he implemented a medical approach to the symptoms he observed. He separated severe illnesses into melancholias (or depression), manias and dementias (which included mental retardation) and suspected the underlying cause of mental illness was a diseased brain. Students of mental illness were encouraged to avoid confusing fact with metaphysical speculations about illness, such as a separation from God. Sympathy for, rather than empathy with, the mentally ill was the most that could be asked of society and the church.

Pinel encouraged social reform in the treatment of the mentally ill based on a revised understanding of its causes.[15] He instituted "moral treatment" of the mentally ill, a humane approach to patients who had been treated as less than human up to that time. These persons could benefit from medical treatment and therefore could not simply be isolated. Theologians contributed little to changing society's views about the mentally ill. Rather, these shifting views about the mentally ill were grounded in the humanism of the Enlightenment coupled with a "can do" attitude that evolved from the Renaissance.

Early in the Christian era, sick and weary travelers were cared for in hospitals, most of which were operated by religious orders. The mentally ill were among those cared for in these refuges from the world. But the responsibility for the sick, especially the mentally ill, was transferred from church to state as early as the 1700s. By that time in Europe, cities were building charity hospitals and asylums. In England privately operated asylums, smaller than the large Continental institutions, were available to treat the mentally ill, particularly those from the upper classes.

In medicine, an emphasis on brain pathology, the neuropsychiatric approach, became the dominant approach to mental illness during the nineteenth century. Though the works of many scientists, such as the biologist Charles Darwin, the psychologist Ivan Pavlov and neuroanatomists such as Camillo Golgi and Ramon y Cajal, were concerned with neuropsychiatry, the prototype neuropsychiatrist was Emil Kraeplin (1856-1926). Like Pinel before him, Kraeplin was an unbiased and persistent observer of the symptoms of the patients under his care. He was the first to differentiate dementia praecox (schizophrenia) from manic-depressive illness, basing this distinction on the outcome of the illness. Kraeplin observed that a patient rarely recovered from dementia praecox but might recover completely from manic-depressive illness.

Kraeplin's work inspired our modern empirical diagnostic system, the *Diagnostic and Statistical Manual of Mental Disorders*.[16] This system bases diagnosis on observable phenomena such as symptoms and outcome rather than theories of causation, including those that blame disordered relations with others or with God and other metaphysical concepts. Yet Kraeplin embraced a nihilistic attitude toward the value of therapies.[17] The psychoanalyst Franz Alexander believed that Kraeplin's contributions to classification "succeeded in bringing into sporadic accumulation of clinical observation a system of distinct disease entities that has stood up remarkably well into the present era. Unfortunately his systematization eventually hindered the deeper understanding of mental disturbances."[18] I agree with Alexander and discuss this further in chapter three.

Interest in Emotional Suffering Emerges Within the Church

Some American Christian leaders during the later nineteenth century grappled with the healing of more severe emotional suffering, but these persons were on the fringe of mainstream Protestant Christianity. Mary Baker Eddy came in contact with the hypnotic techniques of Phineas Quimby for "healing of the mind."[19] Eddy then led a crusade that eventually resulted in the establishment of Christian Science, a movement that encompassed both faith and healing. Though Christian Science never became a mainline Protestant denomination, Eddy's belief that God's healing would restore wholeness to the soul of the mentally ill has reemerged in evangelical and Pentecostal approaches to emotional healing today. Specifically, Christian Science claims the predominance of will over human nature. This approach to healing was more individualistic than previous approaches of the church. As Christian Science denied empirical evidence, however, there was no opportunity for dialogue between its adherents and the empirical psychiatrists of the nineteenth century.

Two secular writers helped shape a more sophisticated and socially aggressive approach to emotional suffering by the church. William James (1842-1910) contributed perhaps the most important statement of nineteenth-century thought relevant to the dialogue between religion and psychiatry.[20] James was one of the founders of modern empirical psychology, and therefore his interest in religion is important to understanding the conversation of the twentieth century.

James, as an experimental psychologist, took a live-and-let-live approach to religion. A pragmatist and empiricist rooted in a liberal Protestant background, James described in detail religious conversions and their psychological benefit in his popular book *The Varieties of Religious Experience*. He concluded that though religion is beyond reason, the unity of religious testimonies leaves open the possibility that religious beliefs may be true. James was not concerned with proving (or disproving) the reality of God.

Perhaps his most important contribution to the conversation between psychiatry and Christianity was his assertion of the right of the individual to believe beyond the evidence. Making every choice based solely on the weight of objective data, for James, is impossible when real-life decisions are forced on people. Therefore the choice of faith is not an unreasonable choice. James thus accommodated faith in his psychology. Faith to James, however, is individualistic, not dependent on the faith community, or God for that matter.

Another nineteenth-century perspective that shaped the interaction between Christianity and psychiatry during the twentieth century was the philosophy of positivism. This line of thought has continued as a hidden but central theme in Protestant theology. Positivism was based on the work of Auguste Comte.[21] Comte believed that society must pass through theological and metaphysical stages to approach its proper goal—a positive, scientific stage. These stages include explanations of experiences attributed first to the gods, later to general abstractions and finally to factual observation. As intellect develops, altruism will triumph over egoism and a religion of humanity will emerge. Rather than worship the God of Abraham, Isaac and Jacob, positivists would worship the famous artists and scientists who have advanced the culture of humankind. At the end, however, each person is responsible to her or his own conscience.

Positivism, based on the conviction that society is progressing to perfection, lost its impetus during the early twentieth century. Europe was moving inevitably toward World War I, and the lives of many Europeans were anything but positive. Minority groups, such as the Czechs, the Poles, the Serbs and the Croats, were expressing discontent with their plight. Realism, pessimism and protest pervaded the literature of the age, revealing the dark side of humanity.

Émile Zola portrayed this awareness in his many novels during the latter nineteenth century. He viewed humanity as selfish, greedy, driven by base desires and not particularly bright. Thomas Hardy's antiheroes were cruel, self-centered or at best tragic. Concurrently, in Vienna a young physician, Sigmund Freud, began to explore the deepest thoughts of his patients through his psychoanalytic methods. He developed the theory that the behaviors and thoughts of women and men derive from the drive for sexual satisfaction or the death instinct, as opposed to more noble drives or instincts. Freud therefore provided a psychological framework for understanding the dark thoughts and behaviors expressed as Europe approached World War I. Freud also opened the door for a conversation between psychiatry and Christianity, since his theory derived from understanding the person in context of his or her social, cultural (and religious) background.

Freud Initiates the Conversation

How did Sigmund Freud initiate a conversation between Christianity and psychiatry? Why wasn't Freud dismissed outright by his Christian contemporaries? Given the questionable efficacy of psychoanalytic therapy, how did psychoanalytic theory affect social and cultural thoughts as profoundly as it did, let alone psychiatric theory?

Freud, born in 1856 in Freiberg to a middle-class Jewish family, was encouraged by his family to respect his culture but not necessarily Judaism. Though Freud's father came from a Hasidic background, he abandoned the traditional beliefs and stringent practices of Judaism. Nevertheless, Freud was exposed frequently to the Hebrew Scriptures in his household and was particularly interested in culture and religion as well as the prevailing scientific optimism of the later nineteenth century.

Sigmund Freud dramatically changed the field of psychiatry. He was firmly rooted in the neuropsychiatry of the nineteenth century and never abandoned the theory that mental actions could be reduced to biological mechanisms. But he developed a form of psychiatric diagnosis and treatment that diverged dramatically from the practices of psychiatrists working in nineteenth-century asylums.

His new method of exploration and healing was psychoanalysis. This psychiatric treatment permitted a doctor to explore the deepest recesses of the mind through techniques such as free association and dream interpretation. Patients could discover the conscious and unconscious dynamic forces controlling their behavior through the guidance of an analyst. The advent of psychoanalysis moved the practice of psychiatry, in large part, from the asylum to the consulting room. Freud's patients were primarily the bourgeoisie, and their problems did not always result in seriously disordered behavior that would demand isolation from society. Freud introduced the world to the psychopathology of everyday life. He also introduced the importance of relationships, real and perceived, in the development of psychopathology. He spoke not only to other doctors but also to the public, using a language understood by both the professional and the nonprofessional, the pastor and the parishioner. His theories had intuitive appeal, and therefore he opened the door for a conversation between theologians and psychiatrists about the nature, function and healing of the soul.

Educated as a physician and neuropathologist, Freud was attracted early in his career to the work of Jean-Martin Charcot in Paris. Through the use of hypnotism, Charcot uncovered thoughts and behaviors in his patients which were hidden during the usual doctor-patient interactions. Charcot demonstrated the unconscious, and Freud undertook to explain it: hypnotism revealed psychopathology in everyday people. Freud's easily read and logical writings introduced the unconscious to the public at large. He brought psychiatry from the asylums to polite society. Freud himself suffered periodic mood swings, episodes of anxiety and an inclination toward gloomy introspection. He therefore engaged in a lifelong self-analysis and encouraged therapists, as well as patients, to explore their unconscious as the source of unexplained sentiments and behaviors.

Psychoanalytic theory was intuitive and attractive to Christians because of the ties between psychoanalysis and Christianity. These ties included the necessity of integrating one's personal story; deliverance from guilt; and confessional exposure of one's darkest thoughts and deeds. Both the pastor and the psychoanalyst were interested in the story of the individual's life, a story of relations in context. For the Christian the context was biblical narratives; for the psychoanalyst it was the dominant myths of society. For example, John Bunyan's *Pilgrim's Progress* was at once the generic story of the unique sacred journey of a man through a difficult life in relation to God and others and the story of personal guilt, internal and interpersonal conflict, catharsis and ultimate healing.[22] Both psychoanalysis and Christianity focused on guilt as the central problem of humankind and release from guilt as the key to healing. Confession to a sympathetic, understanding and confidential confessor was central to healing on the couch and in the church.

Freud, like James, did not deny or overlook the centrality in humankind of relationship with a perceived higher being. Freud, however, challenged Christians regarding their traditional beliefs. He was convinced that religion had no objective validity, that one could find no evidence of a transcendent reality, and therefore religious beliefs and experiences derived solely from human needs and desires.[23] Freud challenged Christians to rethink the sacred Christian story and thereby shook the foundations of Christian beliefs. God, according to Freud, was the longed-for father toward whom humans had, at best, ambivalent feelings. The desire to kill the father (God) resulted in guilt, which had to be expiated through sacrifice (the death of Jesus on the cross). Christianity was therefore a collective neurosis based on suppression and the renunciation of natural instinctive impulses. Christians grounded in the fundamentals of their faith could not tolerate such an interpretation.

Freud also challenged the life story of individual Christians. Psychoanalysis, the treatment for emotional problems developed by Freud, is based on telling and retelling one's life story, leaving not even the most insignificant event, relationship or thought a secret from the therapist. By retelling these stories persons would uncover their own perceived evil (sexual) intentions and the perceived evil (sexual) behavior of their previously idealized parents. Christians, who viewed their corporate history as sacred and their personal histories as innocent and nurturing, reacted violently to this challenge.

Freud did not consider Christianity an aid to healing emotional pain. He assumed religion had no validity and rejected any idea of a transcendent reality.[24] Given his philosophical background, Freud's application of psychoanalytic theory to religion could only conclude that religious experience, ideas and rituals were the result of a perverted attempt to resolve internal conflict and deflect unconscious drives.

Yet Freud's attitude toward religion was complex and conflicted; he described himself as a "completely godless Jew."[25] His antipathy toward religion was directed especially toward Christianity. Late in his life, when Freud was urged to flee the Nazi influence in Austria, he is said to have responded that the true enemy was not Germany but religion, the Roman Catholic Church.[26] He reserved his highest contempt of human nature for the Christian Aryan variety of humankind. His feeling originated in part from an experience his father had. Walking along the street in a new fur cap, his father encountered a Christian who knocked off the cap and said, "Jew, off the sidewalk." His father meekly complied, stepping off to retrieve his cap. Freud faulted his father for not being a strong man who would fight back, and he harbored negative feelings toward Christianity thereafter.[27]

Yet Freud's attack on religion, and specifically Christianity, was not primarily personal. Freud was influenced by theories of physical illness prevalent during the nineteenth century, especially the theory of the physician Ludwig Buchner.[28] Buchner's book, translated *Force and Matter,* went through more than twenty editions and became the militant bible of the scientific-materialistic view of the world. The world as a whole, including the mind, can be explained solely by the activity of materials and their forces, according to Buchner. Therefore God is superfluous. Freud approached the workings of the mind from the perspective of material forces, and despite the broad-ranging psychological, social and existential pronouncements made during his later career, he always viewed himself as a neuropsychiatrist.

Freud was also influenced by the German philosopher Ludwig Feuerbach (1804-1872).[29] To Feuerbach religion is a projection of human qualities into an object of worship; God was created by humankind, not the other way around. Only when these projections are withdrawn and atheism accepted can human limitations and possibilities be accurately assessed. The appropriate object of worship for Feuerbach is humanity. Freud openly avowed that he acquired from Feuerbach and his successors the essential arguments for his personal atheism: "All I have done—and this is the only thing that is new in my exposition—is to add some psychological foundation to the criticisms of my own predecessors."[30]

Freud viewed religion as "nothing but psychology projected to the external world":[31]

A personal God is, psychologically, nothing other than an exalted father. Religiousness is to be traced to the small human child's long-drawn-out helplessness in need of help; and when later in life he perceives how truly forlorn and weak he is when confronted with the great forces of life, the adult feels his condition as he did in childhood, and attempts to deny his own dependency by a regressive revival of the forces which protected his infancy.[33]

Freud's view of religion can be simplified as follows. Most people need and desire religion to cope with their fears of the impersonal power of nature. Therefore, religion takes upon itself the form of a universal neurosis and has its origin in the father complex; belief in God is nothing more than a belief in a magnified father. All religious dogmas are illusions that cannot be proved. As scientific knowledge advances, the need of humankind for religious dogma will diminish. Religion will ultimately be replaced by science, as there will no longer be a need for religion.

These views opened Freud to criticism from both his psychiatric colleagues and Christian theologians. Though these critics were not necessarily opposed to the basic theories of psychoanalysis, they believed that Freud wandered from the scientific base of his theoretical contributions when pronouncing such broad negative views of religion. For the practice of psychoanalysis is interpersonal in essence and renders the therapist a soul doctor, a doctor concerned with the person in relation to others and to the transcendent.

The Conversation with Freud

Though Freud was ardently antireligious, he was rigidly orthodox about psychoanalysis. When disciples of Freud met with him, corresponded with him and discussed his theories, divergent views naturally arose. Freud opposed virtually any challenge to his theory. Conflicts with his early followers therefore arose. One of the earliest and probably the most severe of these conflicts was between Freud and Carl Jung.

Jung, the son of a Protestant minister, was an early member of the inner circle of psychoanalysts. His major contribution to psychiatry was the differentiation of personality types; he described the distinction between the introvert and the extrovert. He also explored the relationship between what he considered universal patterns in the unconscious, or archetypes, and their projections and representations in art, myth and religion.

These inborn, a priori archetypes were used to help explain humankind's relations with the outer world. Archetypes are intuitions that can be interpreted as intuitions of religion. To become mature and unite these collective aspects of personality, the unconscious aspects must merge with the specific aspects of personality resulting from conscious experience. Unlike the personal unconscious of Freud, which is unique to the individual, Jung's universal, or collective, unconscious is inherited by individuals from their culture. Actualization of human potential rests in assimilating or integrating these unconscious contents.[34] Symbols are incorporated by persons to help express and integrate their unconscious.

The split between Jung and Freud emerged partially because of personal conflicts. Freud doubted Jung's loyalty, yet Jung's theories in and of themselves would have been enough to precipitate a split. The two men certainly diverged in their views of religion and its value to humankind. It was a loss to psychiatry and religion that they did not engage in a more extensive conversation regarding their differences.

Early in his career, Jung's views about religion were similar to Freud's in that he perceived God as a projection of the unconscious. Jung later expanded his idea of God and religion as not only projection but also as indispensable symbols that express and encourage the development of psychic wholeness.[35] Persons in all modern societies, despite their individual development, share the uncertainty and disillusionment associated with life dominated by materialism and threatened by the potential of science and technology. For Jung, a technological civilization devoid of those symbols which assist in integrating the human psyche will undermine emotional well-being. In contrast, Freud believed that demythologizing the symbols of religion would free the individual and promote well-being.

Toward the end of his life, Jung wrote extensively of the second half of the life cycle. He concluded that a comprehensive religious system is virtually essential for integrating one's life story near the end of life: "Among all my patients in the second half of life . . . there has not been one whose problem in the last resort was not that of finding a religious outlook on life."[36]

Freud, in contrast, wrote little about later life and the psychological tasks necessary for emotional growth beyond adolescence. Perhaps a stimulus from Jung, if they had maintained contact, would have encouraged Freud to expand his theory to encompass later life. Perhaps such an expansion would have forced him to reconsider the role of religion in adult development, the importance of the religious "outlook."

Freud developed and maintained a more amicable friendship and conversation with the Protestant minister Oscar Pfister, who was his devoted disciple and a strong proponent of psychoanalysis. Yet Pfister did not hesitate to challenge Freud's assumptions regarding religion. Their ongoing correspondence for nearly twenty years was preserved by Freud's daughter Anna.[37] According to Pfister, religion and religious rituals are not solely projections of the unconscious and do not emerge only from the emotionally unhealthy or the immature. Despite the propensity of Christians to engage in wishful thinking about the future, especially the afterlife, even Jesus dismissed the idea of simply waiting for eternal life after death. Rather, Jesus emphasized that the highest ideal is the kingdom of God on this earth, a kingdom realized through the practice of the highest ethical and religious qualities. Religious dogmas are based on reason, not impulse and wishes. Pfister attacked Freud's disbelief head on. "Disbelief is, after all, nothing but a negative belief."[38] Freud's outright dismissal of the possibility of a transcendent God could not be based on anything other than his "belief" in the god of science. Science, Pfister argued, cannot adequately describe the whole person and lacks the ability to explain love and will among persons.[39]

It is remarkable that Freud and Pfister maintained their conversation, as their beliefs were so opposed. One could speculate that the physical distance between Freud and Pfister and the fact that the majority of their discourse was written rather than oral contributed to Freud's willingness to maintain this warm personal friendship. Freud may not have perceived Pfister as a threat to the core dogma of psychoanalysis, a threat he clearly perceived from others in the original inner circle, such as Jung. Pfister also did not challenge the basic tenets of Freud's theories, only the elaborations on religion. Regardless, the result was a rich correspondence between two men who believed differently but who understood each other's views well and welcomed a friendly debate. This debate benefited the development of both psychiatry and Christian theology. Pfister forced Freud to reconsider the atheistic assumptions that were the foundation of his theories about religion, and Freud, in turn, helped shape Pfister's theology in light of psychoanalytic theory.

The Conversation After Freud Among Psychiatrists

Following Freud's death in 1939, the conversation between religion and psychoanalysis continued for at least three decades. For example, the psychoanalyst Gregory Zilboorg joined the conversation between psychiatry and religion during the 1950s. Having converted to Catholicism after his psychiatric training, he wrote *Psychoanalysis and Religion,* emphasizing Freud's ambivalence regarding religious beliefs (a point later expanded by Hans Küng, the Catholic theologian).[40] First, Zilboorg questioned Freud's use of the idea of illusion in describing religion, noting that illusion does not necessarily imply unreality. The human psyche is not the measure of religious truth, since the distortion of truth can occur as easily as the manufacture of falsehood. Zilboorg also challenged Freud regarding the role of conscience in emotional health. For Freud, the superego is an evil that only captivates the natural drives of an individual. These drives are best moderated by an ego firmly rooted in reality, a reality with no room for a punitive God. In contrast, Zilboorg believed that the development of a healthy conscience or superego will lead to integration and maturity, not slavery to one's past.

Zilboorg encouraged a conversation between psychoanalysts and theologians:

> There are a number of earnest religious thinkers who are preoccupied with problems vital to religious life and the life of religion: aggression; ambivalence; the constant clash between love and hate; aesthetic dedication; the contemplative life; moral issues in personal, social and public life; and the relations of the emotions to the problem of will and reason. A number of devout scholars are busy restudying these problems with the utmost care, intellectual honesty, and profound faith. The aid of the added insight which psychoanalysis provides them proves invaluable

both to the further development of religious scholarship and the deeper understanding of the faith.[41]

The devout scholars referred to by Zilboorg were a group of Catholic and Protestant theologians who were thoroughly acquainted with Freud's psychoanalysis. They had recognized the value of his techniques of inquiry for greater understanding of human behavior while recognizing the limitations of his theories.

Karl Menninger joined the conversation from a different perspective. Menninger was probably the best-known psychiatrist in the United States during the mid-twentieth century. In his 1973 book *Whatever Became of Sin?* Menninger summed up his concern about the disappearance of the word *sin* from our language and the shift of responsibility for evil. He bemoaned the apathy of society and did not attribute this apathy to mental illness. Rather, he suggested that mental hygiene results not from reassurance, comforting words or denial of real problems but from deliberate renunciation of apathy and a willingness to take the responsibility for evil. Evil, for Menninger, was neglect of relationships:

> The message is simple. It is that concern is a touchstone. Caring. Relinquishing the sin of indifference. This recognizes acedia as the Great Sin; the heart of all sin. Some call it selfishness. Some call it alienation. Some call it schizophrenia. Some call it egocentricity. Some call it separation.[42]

For Menninger, sin is an abdication of responsibility that derives from "a loss of nerve, a loss of direction, erosion from culture, confusion of thought exhaustion."[43] Yet sin for Menninger is not specific sinful acts requiring specific acts of penance. Attitudes must be changed in order to confront sin. Religion is a source for changing these attitudes.

Christians Respond

Freud directly challenged Christians, for he felt compelled to explore and explain Christian lifestyles and the apparent security of Christians in their beliefs. Why did Christians live as they did? Why did they willingly deny themselves pleasures, especially sexual pleasures? Given that they did, many of them appeared happy and content. To understand the Christian (and persons from all faith traditions), Freud ventured into the social and the cultural, abandoning the more narrow neuropsychiatric tradition.[44] Psychiatry grounded solely in biology was exchanged for speculation about the unconscious, subconscious, subliminal mind. In other words, Freud became a doctor of the soul and necessarily initiated a conversation with those interested in the relations of persons with God and the community.

The writings of Zilboorg and Menninger from within psychiatry dovetailed with the writings of well-known Christian theologians such as Paul Tillich and Richard and Reinhold Niebuhr in the middle of the twentieth century. Menninger was thoroughly familiar with the writings of Tillich and Reinhold Niebuhr and quoted the following passage by Tillich to substantiate his own position:

> Have the men of our time lost a feeling of the meaning of sin? Do they realize that sin does not mean an immoral act, that 'sin' should never be used in the plural, and that not our sins, but rather our sin is the great, all-prevailing problem of our life? To be in the state of sin is to be in the state of separation. Separation may be from one's fellow men, from one's own true self and/or from his God.[45]

Tillich, rather than attempting to Christianize psychiatry, sought to place psychiatry into a broader anthropological and philosophical context. On the whole, Tillich was positive toward pyschoanalytically oriented psychiatry.[46] He specifically believed that Freud conceptualized human nature and its contradictions accurately and recognized the estrangement of humankind.[47] Yet Tillich also recognized the more extensive implications of psychoanalytic theory, as did Pfister, Zilboorg and Menninger. Tillich disentangled neurotic and existential guilt, recognizing the contribution of psychiatry to the healing of neurotic guilt but avoiding the temptation to cover real, existential guilt with analytic theory.[48]

> Man, as finite freedom, is free within the contingencies of his finitude. Though within these limits he is asked to make of himself what he is suppose to become, to fulfill his destiny, in every act of moral self-affirmation man contributes to the fulfillment of his destiny, to actualization of what he potentially is.[49]

Tillich's analogy for seeking God (Being itself) is a courageous journey fraught with anxiety. Existential anxiety comes from fear of the limits of life and death, an anxiety that cannot be relieved by psychoanalysis or medication. Tillich criticized Freud and his followers for impinging blatantly on the realm of theology. Any theory asserting that religion is simply a projection must take responsibility for judging the evidence to determine whether there is something beyond the projection.[50] God is not just "out there," but neither is a relationship with God meaningless.

Tillich's long-time colleague and contemporary at Union Theological Seminary in New York, Reinhold Niebuhr, paralleled Tillich in his cultural and sociological views of the interaction between religion and psychiatry. Niebuhr's challenge to psychiatry was different, however. He recognized the pervasiveness of Freud's views of human nature within Western culture and accepted Freud's assessment of the potential of humankind for destructiveness.[51] For Niebuhr, humankind is inherently sinful, with pride and egotism signs of the Fall. The tragedy is that humankind cannot conceive of its ability to transcend itself yet can conceive transcendence. This leads to anxiety, which, in turn, leads us to try to be more than we can be. Though responsible to God by virtue of freedom of will, there is a most ungodly aspect to human nature that affects all human actions. Prolonged social progress is virtually impossible, for individual imperfections were compounded in society.

The discouragement of many intellectuals following World War I about humankind's social progress was no better manifested than in the writings of Niebuhr:

> Individual men may be moral in the sense that they are able to consider interests of others, other than their own, in determining problems of conduct and are capable, on occasion, of preferring the advantages of others to their own. They are endowed by nature with a measure of sympathy and consideration for their kind . . . but all these achievements are more difficult, if not impossible, for human societies and social groups.[52]

Like Freud, Niebuhr viewed humans, even those pursuing the most noble of goals, as basically self-seeking.[53]

According to Niebuhr, Freud did not understand that human nature, even the unconscious seeking of gratification, extends beyond the biological individual. As did Tillich, Niebuhr emphasized the existential anxiety afflicting humankind:

> It is not repression that creates anxiety; it is there first and creates repression. If Freud could have realized how basic a component of human freedom anxiety is, and how little it has to do with external 'danger', it would have become apparent that all the aberrations with which he deals are not the consequence of the repressions of his 'superego' but arise out of the very character of human freedom.[54]

For Niebuhr, there is something about human nature that cannot be reduced to the biological.

Niebuhr also did not believe Freud understood the self-reflective and self-representational self; a psyche consisting of the ego, superego and id neglects the self. The self is created and internalized in dialogue, especially with others.[55] Niebuhr labeled this self the human spirit, the source of existential anxiety that seeks after the transcendent other. Humans have the capacity to transcend self and, because they are free, are capable of sin, including the sin of focusing on self in the effort to decrease the inherent anxieties of human existence.[56] Niebuhr therefore did not emphasize the individual self but the self within a community, a dialogue that can grow and develop or become perverted.

Niebuhr's brother H. Richard Niebuhr also contributed to the conversation between Christian theology and psychiatry from the perspective of self in community.[57] Specifically, he focused on narrative and its importance to the individual Christian and the church. He recognized a healthy tension between internal and external history, a topic expanded in chapter four. Individual life events are not isolated phenomena but occur within a social context. Humankind has, at best, partial knowledge of this context. The goal of the psychiatrist is to assist patients in understanding their social interactions in context more objectively by commenting on and interpreting these interactions. In like manner, the Christian within the community of the church is forced to accept the external views of self derived from the congregation in which he or she participates. As Robert Burns suggests:

> Oh wad some power the giftie gie us

To see ourself as others see us![58]

To have others communicate what they see when they consider one's life from the outside is to grow within a community. Every reflection of self, such as occurs in psychoanalysis, can be incorporated into the sense of self and therefore can enhance and expand the self. The Christian within the congregation will learn that no external view is absolute "truth" but there is some truth in all views.

Christianity, according to Richard Niebuhr, should likewise appraise its external life rather than focus solely on its inner life. The interpretation of religion and congregational life by the psychiatrist should give pause to the church, should encourage the church to search itself as a corporate body, even as individuals search themselves. Both the individual Christian and the church must integrate the totality of their lives, honestly evaluating both good and bad. Only then can they appreciate grace. Just as psychoanalysis exposes the good, bad and ugly within the individual in order to free the individual from the oppression of the superego, Christianity brings peace and freedom through grace when both the nature of humankind (which is sinful) and the acts of the individual Christian (sins) are revealed and confessed before God by the church and the self. Psychoanalysis and Christian confession require life reviews for the purpose of assisting each person to live within human history and yet maintain freedom from that history.

Richard Niebuhr took this thesis a step further when he described the revelation of God.[59] God revealed himself in history as a self. If a Christian is to know God, he or she must be known by him and therefore know the self as it is reflected in the nature of God. That is, Christians must evaluate themselves through the reflection of God's penetration of self in the conversation between God and humankind. Again, the parallels between this process and psychoanalysis are striking, for the analyst (like God) is, at best, a mirror to the patient to encourage evaluation of self through the penetration of the relationship.

Since the advent of psychoanalysis by Freud, psychoanalysts have increasingly focused on self-psychology and thereby joined theologians, such as the Niebuhrs, in an emphasis on the self and society. Analysts such as

Heinz Kohut led psychoanalysis at mid-twentieth century from focus on the Oedipus complex to a focus on the maturation of the self.[60] The major problem afflicting most persons seeking psychotherapy, according to Kohut, is not conflicts but a deficit in the structure of the self. The task of the therapist is to assist the patient in developing from an infantile state of fragility and fragmentation to a cohesive and stable identity in adulthood. This task is to be accomplished as the therapist becomes a mirror to the patient and empathically adapts to the individual needs of the patient.

Protestant theologians attempted to understand and incorporate psychoanalytic psychiatry into a more informed theology while restraining psychiatry from following Freud's identification of all religion with projection and neurosis. This attempt is reflected in the writings of a philosopher of the early 1970s, Paul Ricoeur.[61] Ricoeur encourages his readers to test their faith in the face of Freud's theories. Though he admits that human beings are quick to project their own fears and conflicts into religious symbolism, he criticizes Freud and his followers for their reductionistic view of religion. Rather than abandoning our immature dependency on religious figures such as Jesus, the goal of psychoanalysis, and indeed maturity, is to find a healthy expression of these needs in our religious attachments. Humans learn to abandon early immature attachments and to substitute the mature, ethical and universal attachments characteristic of the Christian religion.

Ricoeur reflects the trend in modern theology to utilize psychiatric theories but not to stimulate conversation between psychiatry and Christianity. Rather, he applies psychoanalysis as hermeneutics. He defines hermeneutics as "the theory of the rules that preside over . . . the interpretation of a particular text or of a group of signs that may be viewed as a text."[62] Hermeneutics, according to Ricoeur, is structured by a fundamental opposition. A hermeneutics of belief that aims to find meaning in the text by the reader is found at one end. At the other is a hermeneutic suspicion, which reduces and demystifies the text, stripping it of its illusions. On the surface, psychoanalysis is of the latter variety, yet Ricoeur suggests that psychoanalysis can be a hermeneutic of restoration.[63] Ricoeur does not search psychoanalytic theory for empirically testable hypotheses but rather searches psychoanalytic writings to learn what they teach the philosopher/theologian about culture and destiny, that is, persons in relationship. "A meditation on Freud's work has the advantage of revealing that work's broadest aim . . . a reinterpretation of all psychical productions pertaining to culture, from dreams, through art and morality, to religion."[64]

A common characteristic of Tillich, the Niebuhrs and Ricoeur has been their attempt to integrate psychiatry and religion but not to bend psychiatric theory to accommodate religious practice. They were not interested in the pragmatics of psychiatric practice. None asked psychiatry to adopt a specific religious doctrine. None required psychiatrists to convert their patients to the Christian faith. They did, however, encourage psychiatry to create a more philosophically sound and theologically accommodating attitude toward Christians who seek psychiatric care.

The value of this conversation between psychiatrists like Zilboorg and Christian theologians like Reinhold Niebuhr was that both wished to develop a philosophy that would encompass the neuropsychiatric and sociocultural aspects of humankind. Few were so naive to believe that psychiatry could be practiced, that the emotionally suffering could be healed and that harmony could exist between Christianity and psychiatry unless basic philosophical issues are addressed. Some psychiatrists felt compelled to understand their patients in the context of the Christian community, while these Christian theologians recognized the necessity to be well-versed in psychiatric theory. Yet the attempt to reconcile the theories of psychiatry with Protestant theology was difficult.

During the 1960s and into the early 1970s, the conversation evolved into a debate. Specifically, evangelical Christians such as Jay Adams (see below) challenged psychiatry, especially psychoanalytic psychiatrists, as anti-Christian and warned Christians not to seek help from psychiatrists. The debate was less a challenging intellectual debate than a flexing of the muscles of the ever more powerful evangelical thrust. Paradoxically, the debate was more secure for both psychiatrists and Christians, because the positions taken were so radically opposed that little incentive for meaningful conversation, much less reconciliation, emerged. Prior to and during the debate, however, a group of practical theologians, the theologians of pastoral care, joined the conversation.

Clinical Pastoral Education

The most visible remnant of this conversation between Christian theologians and psychiatrists is clinical pastoral education (CPE). The clinical tradition of pastoral care that began during the 1920s was strongly influenced by Freudian psychoanalysis.[65] Anton Boisen began, in 1925, to train seminary students at Worcester State Hospital in Massachusetts. Boisen envisioned the emergence of a new field of specialists:

> Instead of allowing the psychiatrist to remain the exclusive keeper of the lower regions, I am hoping and laboring for the day when the specialist in religion will be able with his help to go down to the depths of the grim abyss after those who are capable of responding, those in whom some better self is seeking to come to birth.[66]

After specializing in the study of the psychology of religion at Union Theological Seminary, Boisen experienced a sudden psychotic episode that required him to be hospitalized as a psychiatric patient. Thereafter he was convinced that practical exposure to the mentally ill would clarify and provide examples of the theological and ethical dimensions of the Christian faith. Theology would be internalized through this exposure. The metaphor that emerged to explain this internalization was *insight,* an insight easily transferred from psychoanalysis to pastoral care. Insight and understanding, in turn, will promote tolerance—acceptance of feelings, the body and sexuality. In addition, this insight will overcome the rigidity and condemnation inherent in the more conservative Protestant mindset. Pastoral counselors will empathize with persons rather than emphasize the conventions and rules of the faith tradition. In other words, Boisen wished to change the relationship of persons with emotional problems and their faith community through a reinterpretation of the teachings of that community.

Howard Clinebell, a prototypical pastoral counselor, lists five central ideas based on Boisen's approach which played a decisive role in shaping pastoral counseling during the 1940s and 1950s. These ideas are closely associated with psychoanalysis: a structured interview (the classic fifty-minute hour of the psychoanalyst), a client-centered method (nondirective counseling), insight as the central goal of counseling, the concept of unconscious motivation and the childhood roots of adult behavior.[67] Boisen not only was comfortable with the basic premises of psychoanalytic therapy, he translated them directly into a model of counseling that could be adopted by the pastor of a church. Yet he did little to expand them based on Christian theology.

The emergence of CPE was not uniformly accepted in the Protestant churches, even by more liberal Protestant theologians. The theology of adjustment that undergirded CPE was antithetical to a genuine religion, according to Tillich. True theology does not adjust its values to the values of the dominant culture.[68] Nevertheless, adjustment and the demand for acceptance of reality in religious growth, coupled with a recognition of innate freedom, dominated as the paradigm for pastoral counseling.

Rollo May, a pastor turned psychologist, was the prototypical theological realist. May proposed that human life is marked by a healthy tension between freedoms and the demand of reality.[69] Insight is translated into a capacity to trust in reality, and faith is redefined as trust. Reality is, in large part, the actual relation between a person and her or his culture.

This theology of faith as trust, gained through insight and the therapeutic relationship, gave way to a somewhat different orientation among pastoral counselors after World War II. At that time they came under the influence of Carl Rogers. Rogers was especially appealing given the trends of this era. Cultural trends moved away from legalism toward a preoccupation with psychology, postwar affluence and an ethic of self-realization.[70] William Glasser has described these trends as the transition of America to an identity society, no longer preoccupied with acquiring the necessities of living but concentrating on introspection and the search for personal identity.[71] Pastoral counselors were ideally situated not only to heal damaged emotions but also to enhance psychological development, unleash hidden potentials and find personal identity.

Rogers was most positive about human nature and human potential. He saw virtually no limits to the capacity of persons with distorted or conflicted personalities, as long as the therapist did not interfere with personal growth. He therefore developed an approach to counseling based on nondirective interaction with patients. Among the most damaging interventions made by a therapist, he believed, is the giving of advice. Through his nondirective method, he attempted not to change the person but to nurture the person who was existentially there.

The theories of Rogers were at variance with theological realism and the call to adjust to society. Social institutions, including the church, were viewed as impositions on human freedom and dignity.[72] Rogerian counseling had the paradoxical effect of isolation of faith from community. Here Rogers followed the lead of the psychoanalyst and popular writer Erich Fromm.

Fromm, who encouraged the expression of one's unique individuality born of love to affirm self and others, was also appealing to pastoral counselors.[73] The influence of Rogers and Fromm, especially the nondirective, nonjudgmental therapeutic approach of Rogers, created an atmosphere of thoroughgoing acceptance among pastoral counselors.[74] Pastoral counselors were encouraged to exhibit toward the counselee an attitude of unconditional positive regard. This empathic, nonjudgmental adaptation to the counselee's frame of reference would assure counselees that they were accepted as they were.

Rogerian therapy was also a safe method for those not trained extensively in counseling. The Rogerian counselor would not fall into the trap of giving bad advice or directing attention away from the counselee as long as the attitude of unconditional positive regard was maintained. As described below, it is not surprising that pastoral care under the influence of Rogers gradually separated from the Christian community.

Insight and understanding, as prescribed by Freud, remained central to the counseling techniques employed by the pastoral counselors of the 1950s and 1960s. Nevertheless, Freudian psychology, especially Freudian views of the origin of religious sentiments, had faded to the background, and self-realization and self-actualization ascended to prominence. Theological interest in Freud likewise faded. Theologians such as Reinhold Niebuhr shifted their challenge to Rogers for his excessive optimism about growth and self-realization and the lack of awareness of the impulse toward selfishness inherent in Rogerian theory.

Pastoral counselors, however, followed Rogers.[75] During the late 1950s and 1960s some pastoral counselors and Protestant theologians were having second thoughts about the evolution of pastoral care. The 1960s saw the growth of a variety of therapies and the emergence of the so-called psychological society. A therapeutic vocabulary invaded society with expressions such as "hang loose," "find yourself," "claim your own space" and "do your thing," which cut against the grain of the Christian community. Many pastoral counselors left the institutional church to set up private practices or to take positions in health care facilities.

Others, however, questioned whether true pastoral care could occur outside of the church.[76] Could self-actualization occur outside the context of group and interpersonal relations? This tension regarding pastoral care continues today. Some pastoral counselors expressed more basic concerns, questioning whether the psychological goal of mental health was equivalent to the spiritual goal of growth and salvation. Albert Outler, for example, emphasized the need for theology to check and limit the assumptions of the new psychotherapies. For instance, true self-realization requires self-denial, not self-actualization.[77]

Pastoral counselors also struggled for an identity separate from secular psychotherapists. Some suggested that context defines pastoral care, but context is an abstract concept that did not penetrate to the pastor and the parishioner. Though the American Association of Pastoral Counselors voted in the late 1960s to oppose the private practice of pastoral counseling, or practice outside the context of the church, this did little to stem the tide of pastoral counselors setting up practices next to, or even in partnership with, secular therapists.[78] Pastoral care in large part became indistinguishable from secular therapies popular during the later twentieth century.

Despite the separate training programs, pastoral care today is defined more by its distinctive role than by a unique approach to caring for those suffering emotionally. In other words, the pastoral counselor is a pastor who counsels using methods, for the most part, indistinguishable from those of the secular psychologist. The religious identification of the pastoral counselor is evident in his or her title rather than in the utilization of theology to guide his or her practice. These roles are more likely to be found outside the church than within, in the position of hospital or military chaplain. A hospital chaplain, then, is a pastoral counselor who may be indistinguishable from the secular therapist who consults with patients suffering emotional as well as physical problems.

Perhaps I have overstated the case. Yet pastoral care, despite having rendered much service to the suffering, has stimulated little conversation or debate between psychiatry and Christianity.

The stage was therefore set for a new movement: evangelical Christian counseling. Christian counselors from evangelical backgrounds with professional training were rare before the 1960s. For the Christian counseling movement to firmly establish itself, a unique identity was essential. Pastoral care had claimed the role for mainline Protestant Christianity, even if it did occur outside the institutional church. Freud had little influence over the newer psychotherapies that were widely practiced by psychiatrists and pastoral counselors, and during the 1960s psychiatry moved largely away from Freud. Nevertheless, Freud and what he was perceived to represent became a central focus in establishing the initial identity of evangelical Christian counselors. The "Freud versus God" debate was the metaphor that framed the ascent of evangelical Christian counseling.

Conversation Becomes Debate

Extraordinary persons engaged the conversation between psychiatry and Christianity during the mid-twentieth century. These persons were grounded in their own fields yet well-read and informed across other fields such as history, sociology and anthropology. They were especially knowledgeable as theologians about psychiatry and as psychiatrists about Christian theology. They also spoke to the general public. Educated nonprofessionals could understand the writings of both Freud and Reinhold Niebuhr.

Such breadth of understanding and ability to explain became increasingly difficult to achieve, however, as the knowledge base of each field of study increased and specialization replaced generalism. Some psychiatrists withdrew into psychoanalytic theory as dogma. They now perceived as their mission the freeing of unsophisticated Christians from their archaic and restrictive beliefs, rather than conversing with them. Evangelical Christians retreated to the fundamental security of the Scriptures and launched a frontal attack on what they viewed as the hedonistic, atheistic philosophy of psychoanalytic psychiatry. Battle lines were drawn for many psychiatrists and evangelical Christians during the sixties. The fields of battle were the nature of guilt, Freud's professed atheism, sexual freedom, the truth versus the fiction of one's life story, whether the Christian faith is a strength or a weakness, and whether the psychiatrist or the pastor should be the confessor of the emotionally suffering.

Perhaps another reason psychiatrists and evangelical Christians drew battle lines against one another was their relative positions within society. A. T. Grounds has noted that

> the place occupied by theologians in universities is similar to that occupied by psychiatrists in medicine. Both evoke responses of perplexity or sarcastic joking from their academic colleagues. . . . Both psychiatrists and theologians are faced with the problem of convincing others of the value of what they do.[79]

Psychiatrists and evangelical Christians alike were ridiculed as unsophisticated by their colleagues. A typical response to being undervalued is to displace that perception to another group. (Many of the prejudices in our society have emerged from such displacement.) For this reason and others, conservative evangelical Christians became convenient targets for some psychiatrists, and vice versa.

Psychiatry had encountered problems and undergone change following the halcyon years of psychoanalysis during the first half of the twentieth century. Psychoanalysts were criticized by other medical specialists for refusing to submit their treatment techniques to empirical study. The idea that long hours and many dollars spent on psychoanalysis enhanced patients' emotional well-being or cured their psychiatric disorders was far from proven.

Some psychoanalysts, in turn, challenged Christianity as unscientific mysticism of the uneducated. This challenge to Christianity by psychoanalysts, ostensibly derived from a scientifically based analytic dissection of religion, could have been in part a deflection of the challenges to psychoanalysis from other medical specialties. Regardless, these psychiatrists left no room for Christian beliefs in their prescriptions for healing. They asserted that Christianity undermines the emotional well-being of its adherents. Religions such as Christianity exploit individuals by their institutional character and their ability to control persons and inhibit the free expression of natural drives. Religion also maintains institutional oppression over its adherents by shaping and facilitating the superego's guilt, with all of its detrimental and pathological effects.[80] Religion perpetuates immaturity, both personal and intellectual. There is no compromise. Not only are emotional well-being and psychological maturity incompatible with fundamental Christian beliefs, they are in part an escape from those beliefs. As suggested by Feuerbach a century before, "man's God is MAN. This is the highest law of ethics."[81]

I can testify to this perception by mainstream psychiatry of evangelical Christianity at the time I entered psychiatry. Though I was accepted, most of my colleagues expected that my religious views would change dramatically as I progressed in psychiatric training. If I attempted to engage in a discussion of psychiatry and religion, my questions were dismissed. Some of my fellow trainees could not accept that Sunday was a special day for me and occasionally became angry if I declined an offer to attend a social gathering because of my participation in church activities. Yet these experiences were rare. I was easily incorporated into the Duke community as long as I did not say much about my religious beliefs.

Perhaps the most disturbing aspect of those first years at Duke was not any challenge to my faith but that my faith was dismissed as trivial. I soon learned that as long as I kept quiet about my beliefs, even if others knew, I had no difficulty relating to the faculty or my fellow trainees.

Despite the relatively uncompromising view of some psychoanalysts during the fifties and sixties, other psychiatrists remained open to conversation. Earl Biddle, for example, wrote during the fifties about the integration of psychiatry and religion.[82] He postulated that the rift between psychiatry and religion is based on the materialist terms used by psychiatry to describe human behavior. "It is to be expected that scientific explanations of human behavior in purely materialistic terms will be met by opposition, not only by the clergy, but by everyone concerned about religion."[83] Psychoanalytically oriented psychiatrists approached the problem of guilt as a conflict to be resolved through psychoanalysis that would break the constraints on the natural drives, especially sexual drives. A Christian morality that limits sexual freedom was deemed immature if not pathological.

In general, psychiatrists during the sixties did not frontally attack Christianity but rather viewed it as evidence of emotional immaturity and lack of intelligence. For example, in 1965 Edgar Draper and his colleagues explored the diagnostic value of a religious interview.[84] Though they did not uniformly recommend religious inquiry, they suggested that a patient's religious views could be useful for determining a psychiatric diagnosis. "Unpsychologically minded patients . . . were found especially able to talk about themselves in terms of religious activities or beliefs, whereas they often had been guarded in routine psychiatric interviews." As an example, these authors proposed that one man's conclusion that evil exists in the world because people run away from God and from the Bible's rules and regulations was a compulsive response to guilt over his own destructive impulses. His desire to contribute to peace in the world derived from a phallic preoccupation resulting from his feelings of inadequacy as a man. In other words, this man's faith was not real nor beneficial. His noble goals did not derive from noble motivations.

Carl Christensen, in another paper published during this period, explored Christian conversion.[85] Persons experiencing religious conversion, he said, cannot resolve their guilt and anger through ordinary, healthy means. "Religious beliefs helped to maintain the repression and to support the ego, hence, any challenge to those beliefs is perceived as a threat and must be defended." Conversion was therefore characterized as immaturity and weakness.

The above examples are not typical of psychiatric writings during the 1950s and 1960s. When searching the psychiatric literature during this era, one has difficulty finding overt anti-Christian expressions. Rather, the attitude expressed by psychiatrists simply trivialized the faith of Christians, especially the simple faith of the uneducated, evangelical Christian.

Stephen Carter has captured this modern American attitude toward religion in his book *The Culture of Disbelief.*[86] He suggests that in the name of religious freedom, expression of belief is restricted and trivialized in

American society. For example, a Conservative Jew who enlisted in the army believed he should wear a skullcap under his army cap but was not permitted to do so in the name of religious freedom or the separation of church and state. Religious beliefs are accepted as long as they are not expressed in words or actions toward others of a different persuasion.

The Group for the Advancement of Psychiatry noted in 1947 that psychiatry does not conflict with the morals and ethics of religion but frees persons to assert the morality and ethics that stem from conscious affirmation, reasoned devotion and accepted behavior rather than from a compulsive, fear-based pattern of behavior.[87] This "value-neutral" psychiatry was perceived by evangelical Christians, however, as anything but value-neutral. Instead it was a challenge to their beliefs in the name of acceptance.

The trivialization by psychoanalysts of Christianity was questioned even by secular psychologists. An early challenge to Freudian psychiatry came from within mainline psychology and was quickly picked up by evangelical Christian counselors. O. Hobart Mowrer, a former president of the American Psychological Association, argued that repression of the superego (the conscience) via alignment of the ego with the id results in pathology rather than cure. He went even further and challenged Christians to take up the fight. "Has evangelical religion sold its birthright for a mess of psychological pottage?"[88] Jay Adams, a pastor and a student of Mowrer, concluded that most of the persons he interviewed in mental institutions were there "not because they were sick, but because they were sinful. In counseling sessions, we discovered with astonishing consistency that the main problems people were having were of their own making. Others . . . were not their problem; they themselves were their own worst enemies."[89]

Just as psychiatrists in the 1960s appeared to have little desire to converse with Christians, evangelical Christian counselors, such as Adams, emerged who had little or no desire to converse with psychiatrists. When the subject was the nature of guilt, there was virtually no room for conversation, much less reconciliation.

That the work of counseling should be carried on preeminently by ministers and other Christians whose gifts, training and calling especially qualify and require them to pursue the work, I do not doubt. . . . Medical problems demand close cooperation with the physician (preferably a Christian). Yet, to say all this in no way denies or distracts from the competency of the Christian counselor to counsel. . . . He should see no need, therefore, to defer to a self-appointed caste of men called psychiatrists who have scientifically declared that their province necessarily extends beyond his own.[90]

The target of the evangelical Christian attack on psychiatry was Freud's perceived view of Christianity. Freud did "scientifically declare" that the province of psychiatry extends beyond the brain to the mind and soul of the person, especially in his later writings. For evangelical Christians the conflict was framed as the "Freud versus God" debate. Freud's expressed atheism was the barrier to dialogue. Though Freud and Pfister had carried on a congenial correspondence, the lay perception of Freud did not set a mood for congeniality.[91]

I read the works of Jay Adams while I was in psychiatric training. Unfortunately, his argument shed more heat than light on the conversation I was seeking. I found myself reacting more negatively toward Adams than I reacted toward the psychiatrists who appeared to trivialize my faith. Basically, I read Adams as saying that, beyond drugs, there is no room for a doctor in treating the Christian who experiences emotional suffering. I also reacted to his attack on Freud, which to me, even at that stage of my training, appeared superficial, caustic and nonproductive. A Catholic theologian, Hans Küng, appeared closer to the truth.

Küng attempted to soften the barrier in his 1979 book *Freud and the Problem of God*. Analyzing Freud's atheism, Küng concluded that psychoanalytic theory, despite its overt atheism, contained from the beginning a foundation for considering the spiritual. Many Jews view Freud as a religious person—a view incredible to many evangelical Christians. According to the Talmud, however, if a man denies God but lives according to his precepts, the man is acceptable to God. Therefore many believe that Freud, despite his writings about the neurotic nature of religious beliefs and practices, was in fact religious in his sincerity, his integrity and the persistence of his devotion to his theories and profession.[92]

Psychoanalytic theory, as it evolved through time, was not as antireligious as Freud's writings implied. Freud's disciples, such as Jung and Viktor Frankl, easily shifted the focus of psychoanalytic theory of psychopathology from repressed sexuality to identity and meaning. Psychologists such as Erik Erikson and Rollo May, grounded in psychoanalysis, identified the angst among many Westerners in the middle of the twentieth century as deriving from a sense of emptiness, a concept to which Christian counselors could easily ally themselves.[93] Nevertheless, most evangelical Christian counselors felt the need to mount a counterattack on the perceived atheism and hedonism of psychoanalysis.

Evangelical Christians also had great difficulty, especially during the turbulent 1960s, accepting the implications of Freud's emphasis on sexual freedom. Was it not the self-conscious recognition of their nakedness that signaled the deception of sin for Adam and Eve? Adam and Eve covered their nakedness with fig leaves. Was not the uncovering of sexual desire and pleasure by Freud at the very heart of sin? Freud had taken the issue of sexuality far beyond a freeing of sexual desires. He dared to suggest that the normal development of the innocent child progresses through a stage during which the child feels sexual desires for the parent of the opposite sex coupled with the desire to kill the parent of the same sex, a stage known as the Oedipus complex. Such an interpretation of the innocence of children, the very children whom Jesus had proposed as examples for adults, was not easy to accept by the family-oriented evangelical Christian counselor. If Jesus encouraged "little children [to] come to me . . . for the kingdom of heaven belongs to such as these" (Mt 19:14), then Freud's concept of children could not be tolerated.[94]

According to psychoanalytic theory, the conflicts that result from lack of resolution of the Oedipus conflict and any other arrested or perverted development of the child are resolved as the patient retells his or her life story. The problem of the neurotic is the problem of an inaccurate view of her or his past, which in turn leads to an inaccurate interpretation of the sociocultural past. Christians were also concerned with the individual life story lived within the context of the sociocultural past, that is, religious heritage. The goal of the Christian is to live her or his life story within the larger gospel story. Stanley Hauerwas, in *A Community of Character,* suggests that the Christian community is in fact "story formed."[95] The task of the church is to be the kind of community that tells, and tells correctly, the story of Jesus. Though the story cannot be accurately guaranteed on every historical point, the community must nevertheless carry the story and communicate it with joy.

A fundamental difference existed between views of the story of evangelical Christians and psychoanalysts. For the Christian the larger story is the critical story, and the story of each individual is lived within this larger story. One finds meaning for one's individual life in the story of Jesus. The psychoanalyst, in contrast, encourages patients to challenge the larger story based on a reinterpretation of their individual stories. If the patient loved his mother and wished to kill his father in order to possess the mother sexually, then surely the Christian faith must have arisen from a similar conflict. In *Totem and Taboo* Freud described how this must have happened.[96] The primitive community was dominated by one powerful and violently jealous male who captured women for himself and either drove off or killed all of his rivals, including his sons.

> One day the brothers who had been driven out came together, killed and devoured their father and so made an end of the patriarchal horde. United, they had the courage to do and succeed in doing what would have been impossible for them individually. . . . The violent primal father had doubtlessly been the feared and envied model of each one of the company of brothers: and in the act of devouring him, they accomplished their identification with him and each one of them acquired a portion of his strength.[97]

The Christian doctrine of atonement, for Freud, is a poorly disguised admission of the guilt that derives from this primitive deed. Christ, the Son, represents the guilt through his own sacrifice. The Eucharist becomes symbolic of the original sacrifice that both eliminated the Father and atoned for the guilt. This story of Jesus is far from the treasured story believed by evangelical Christians.

One of the main attractions of psychiatry to me was the opportunity to hear the stories of the people I treated and to possibly help them through a reinterpretation of those stories. Yet I could not accept either the orthodox psychoanalytic view or the superficial view of one's life story. The psycho-analytic view seemed too narrowly focused on sexual development, so the writings of persons such as Rollo May, Viktor Frankl and Erik Erikson were much more in concert with my views of childhood and adult development. The superficial Christian view of the idealized family was equally unacceptable. Life is tough (my own childhood wasn't that pleasant) for Christian and non-Christian alike. Yet learning to tell one's life story seemed central to healing, and hearing that story seemed central to doctoring.

Not only did Freud view the Christian faith as arrested development, he viewed religion as weak. Religion is an opiate (as Karl Marx had also suggested).[98] Religion serves as a conciliation for the injustices of life, encouraging persons to accept their political and socioeconomic status and refuse to challenge those who oppress them.

> A man makes the forces of nature not simply into persons with whom he can associate as he would with his equals—that would not do justice to the over-powering impressions which those forces make on him—but he gives them the character of a father. He turns them into gods, following in this, . . . an infantile prototype.[99]

Evangelical Christians could not tolerate the accusation that they were inherently weak. Are Christians not "soldiers" marching into battle? Is pacifism (where it is embraced) to be equated with impotence? Is the cross to be only a sign of capitulation to evil in the world? Once Christianity's strength and integrity were challenged, Christians could not but retaliate, challenging Freud himself. That Freud was Jewish perhaps facilitated the confrontation, for some Christians greatly fear Jews (a fear that has fueled anti-Semitic views for millennia), believing that ever since the Jews killed Christ, they have been trying to destroy the Christian faith. This blatant prejudice surely contributed to the debate, as the leaders of American psychiatry during the 1960s were predominantly Jewish. In reality psychiatrists have not singled out Christian beliefs for destruction; Freud challenged the foundation of Jewish faith as directly as he challenged Christianity.

From my perspective, Christianity was not so weak that it could not examine itself. Psychoanalysis and the philosophies that form the foundation of Freudian psychoanalysis must be seriously considered by the thoughtful Christian. Freud challenged me to review my beliefs and my faith community. If my reflex was to attack rather than to reflect and converse, then I did not see my faith as worthy of serious thought. I could not live with a mindless Christianity.

Finally, the debate was reduced to pragmatics, or questions as to who is the appropriate confessor. I do not mean "confessor" in the traditional sense of the Catholic Church. Protestant Christianity eliminated the necessity of a confessor and encouraged the Christian to commune directly with God through the divine intermediary, Jesus. The new confessor is the person who helps in the process of emotional catharsis. Both the evangelical pastor and the psychiatrist were asking those who suffered emotionally to confess their innermost feelings. Both promised healing of the emotions.

At the time when Freud began to dominate psychiatry, Christians had previously received psychiatric care, in large part, only for the most severe psychiatric problems. Treatment generally had been within hospitals and with biologically based therapies such as electroshock. Psychotherapy in the office of a psychiatrist was relatively rare until the emergence of psychoanalysis. Until then the pastor had been the natural counselor for the ordinary person experiencing emotional problems. Competition naturally arose between the cloth and couch as evangelical pastors increasingly sought training in secular counseling as a step in professional development.

The debate, though short-lived, was a heated one. When I first considered becoming a psychiatrist in 1969, I stepped into the thick of the battle. My friends in the church of Christ were incredulous. "How can you be a Christian and a psychiatrist at the same time?" "Those psychiatrists will turn you into an atheist." "Psychiatrists can't help you; they will only force you to give up your faith."

The predicted debate never fully materialized. Even as the flames were fanned, they were quenched. Changes were occurring in both psychiatry and Christianity around 1970 which would bring this debate virtually to an end within twenty years. How did this happen? Psychiatrists were quick to forget Freud, Jung, Frankl and Menninger. Psychiatry could not maintain its legitimacy as a medical specialty as long as it kept psychoanalysis at its core. Discoveries of biological mechanisms of disease and the application of technologically sophisticated diagnostic procedures and therapies were the driving forces in medicine by the 1970s. The discovery of penicillin and other medications between World War I and II provided powerful tools to the physician. Therapies proved effective in controlled experiments undergirded the major medical specialties. Advanced technology opened entirely new approaches to diagnosing disease. For example, cardiac catheterization, which became a routine diagnostic procedure during the 1970s, permitted a direct view of the arteries of the heart; coronary bypass surgery brought instant relief to those suffering heart pains. Psychiatry soon followed suit with the rise of neuropsychiatry. Psychiatrists ceased searching for soul.

Christians, for their part, forgot Tillich and the Niebuhrs. Modern evangelical Christian counselors have avoided meaningful discussions of the theological implications of modern psychiatry, especially neuropsychiatry. The remnants of the conversation and debate are hidden away in divinity-school courses on the theory of pastoral care and hermeneutics or in attacks on our anti-Christian culture as a whole, rarely opened up to the Christian sitting in the pew. The Christian instead hears the neuropsychiatrist's promise of a pill to heal all ills and the emerging Christian counseling industry's prescriptive formulas for health, wealth and happiness—calls that complement rather than conflict with one another.

The Comfortable Accommodation

At a time when factions appear to rend the fabric of Western society, a comfortable spirit of accommodation characterizes the current relationship between psychiatry and Christianity. Stephen Jay Gould provides a context for understanding this accommodation when he proposes that religion and evolution can live in harmony because they speak two different languages:

> Science and religion are harmonious because they live in different domains, each of which is important to anyone's full life. Science is an inquiry into the factual state of nature and the explanation of how those facts got that way, and religion is the domain of ethics and values. There is no reason why they should overlap. Any full life needs to consider both

sides. But that is a style of harmony. They are harmonious because they do not conflict.[100]

Such a statement from an evolutionary biologist would shock evangelicals who view evolutionary theory as a direct challenge to the biblical account of creation. Yet these same evangelicals approach the relationship between psychiatry and Christianity as harmonious. Psychiatry and Christianity may now speak different languages, but it is far from certain that they live in different domains and therefore are harmonious.

One Christian counselor echoes this spirit of accommodation when describing the nature of depression: "Depression often has a physical basis. . . . [Medical approaches] help with symptom relief. . . . The non-medical counselor is not qualified to decide whether or not the counselee's physical symptoms are psychologically induced."[101] Though this counselor suggests that the spiritual and the physical overlap, even that spiritual crises may cause physical symptoms, he is ready to defer to the psychiatrist whenever the depression is severe. Virtually all severe depressions are accompanied by physical symptoms. If the depression is severe, it is perceived to be beyond the boundaries of Christian theology and the help of the nonmedical Christian counselor. By implication, severe emotional suffering is also beyond the influence of the Christian community. The healing community cannot minister to persons with severe mental illnesses.

What a paradox! Suicidal thoughts, the most severe of depressive symptoms, cut to the heart of Christian theology perhaps more than psychiatry. Albert Camus said, "There is but one truly serious philosophical problem and that is suicide. Judging whether life is or is not worth living amounts to answering the fundamental question of philosophy."[102]

An episode of severe depression is not the time for the Christian to defer all responsibility to the psychiatrist. At the least, severe depression is the joint responsibility of the cloth and the couch. Severe depression that leads to a suicide attempt by a Christian is a spiritual crisis and requires a conversation between the pastor and the psychiatrist, a coordinated effort between the hospital and the church, not just accommodation.

Psychiatrists and Christians have decided to live and let live when caring for the severely and chronically mentally ill. Christians promise to care for the ancillary theological uncertainty that might be associated with a severe emotional problem, yet psychiatrists care for the *real* problem. Psychiatrists likewise admit dual roles and have even entered "religious uncertainty" as a separate category into their diagnostic system (*Diagnostic and Statistical Manual of Mental Disorders,* 4th ed. [DSM-IV]), a category that, by definition, they defer to the pastor.[103] (See chapter four.)

We are much more likely today to read of the accommodation of Christianity and psychiatry than of their conflicts.[104] For example, John McIntyre, a recent president of the American Psychiatric Association, led a delegation of psychiatrists on a pilgrimage to Salt Lake City, Utah, in 1994. Their goal was to visit Mormon leaders and improve the dialogue between religion and psychiatry. He made a similar pilgrimage in 1993 to visit the pope with a goodwill delegation of psychiatrists. These psychiatrists have declared that the war between psychiatry and religion is at an end and now wave the banner of peace.[105]

From a pragmatic/functional perspective, the cooperation of psychiatrists and Christians, compared to a hostile debate, is good for both patients and practitioners. Nevertheless, the current accommodation is based not on dialogue but on parallel practice. Psychiatry does not inform Christianity, and Christianity does not inform psychiatry. As we enter an era when some suggest that scientific insights into brain function raise the prospect of made-to-order, off-the-shelf personalities, an era during which the antidepressant Prozac has virtually become a cult drug, surely a dialogue is essential if emotional suffering is not to be considered as capable of being simply drugged or thought away.[106] Psychiatry does not appear to be concerned that Christianity has abdicated far too much responsibility to professionals for the care of the severely mentally ill. Christianity does not appear concerned that psychiatry has relegated human nature and conduct, including the spiritual, to brain biology.

Perhaps even more disturbing, both psychiatry and Christianity have only skimmed the surface of the angst that pervades modern Western society. Psychiatrists have drugged and Christians have denied many of the stressors of modern life which cause emotional suffering and drive people away from one another and from their faith traditions. How did this happen? I suggest in the following chapters that both psychiatry and Christianity have abandoned discussion of critical issues most relevant to emotional suffering. They have neglected personal and social history and have spent too little time struggling with the painful realities of our society. Some unholy and unhealthy themes are dominating both psychiatry and Christianity, themes that pervade Western society as a whole. We live in a disturbingly narcissistic society, a society that demands immediate gratification, including the right to emotional well-being as well as self-realization and self-fulfillment. Given modern technology, we believe we need not suffer. If the consumer demands instant relief, both the psychiatrist and the Christian counselor feel compelled to deliver relief.

Anti-intellectualism also pervades both psychiatry and Christianity. "Think pieces," writings that explore the theoretical and philosophical roots of psychiatric illness and treatment, are infrequent in psychiatric literature. When they do appear, they rarely break with current paradigms. Christians, meanwhile, write around rather than through the core issues of mental anguish. Both psychiatry and Christianity have accepted uncritically, to a large extent, the biological reductionism of psychopharmacology.

The task of the psychiatrist should not be primarily to diagnose a particular neuropathological abnormality or select a particular drug to correct a chemical imbalance. Psychiatry is about people's emotional pain and disordered behavior in the context of their life stories, their aspirations, their successes, their failures, their relationships, and the meaning these give to their lives. That is, psychiatry is concerned with soul as well as brain. Christianity is not about instant relief, immediate gratification and the power of positive thinking. Christianity is about living one's life within the context of the story of Jesus. The Christian life is a goal-directed life given meaning by the fullness of the Judeo-Christian heritage, a life that struggles every step of the way, a life that often suffers emotionally. Christianity is about care for emotional suffering through perseverance within a community of care. Christianity is about people living in relationship with other people and God.

Even so, psychiatrists and Christians are less likely to speak with one another of these issues today than in the early or mid-twentieth century. The conversation is infrequent, the debate is ended, and the opportunity for new insights has been temporarily lost. I rarely find someone who asks me today, "How can you be a psychiatrist and a Christian at the same time?" Perhaps they prefer and expect me to live a segmented, and therefore solitary, life in the hospital and the church. Yet I cannot relate to my psychiatric colleagues except as a Christian, nor to my Christian brothers and sisters except as one who practices psychiatry.

3

Psychiatry Loses Its Soul

I *selected psychiatry as a specialty* so I could relate to people. I enjoyed listening to people, learning about their activities, their values, their aspirations, as well as their problems. The experience of seeing 150 patients a day as a primary-care physician in Africa made the luxury of getting to know people my main attraction to psychiatry. I could help people in any specialty, but only in psychiatry could I read the heart and soul of people. And that is exactly what I found in the early 1970s. Today, however, even as I try to know my patients and speak their language, many barriers have arisen between us. I spend less time with my patients, but time constraints are not the only barriers between my patients and me. We are no longer soul mates.

At the middle of the twentieth century, psychiatry spoke to the soul of American society, and society expressed its soul in the language of psychiatry. Virtually every mental struggle or emotional pain was cast into a psychosocial explanatory framework by the community. Even then, however, Americans were becoming more isolated from their communities and viewed their emotional pain as an internal rather than a relational problem.

If we questioned the meaning of life, we probably were experiencing an identity crisis. If we were uncertain about the right or wrong of a behavior, we were experiencing a neurotic conflict. Human problems of living were not viewed as normal variations of the life course of sociocultural relations or as unexpected twists of fate, but rather as the products of internal psychological maladjustments. People could not view themselves as normal, because we all suffered some degree of internal psychological maladjustment. To overcome our maladjustment we needed psychiatry, not other people—a healing of the soul by doctors of the soul. Some critics appropriately expressed concern about the seduction of society by psychiatry, but few denied that psychiatry spoke to the soul of society.

Psychiatry was not only valued as a medical treatment. Psychiatric theory was believed to be of immediate value in virtually every area of society. Vance Packard, in his bestselling book *The Hidden Persuaders,* described a new era of using psychological and psychiatric theories to market billions of dollars of merchandise, services and even political candidates.[1] The concern expressed by Packard and others about how psychiatry had captured the soul of America shows that psychiatry spoke to the needs and struggles of persons at mid-twentieth century. The language and theories of psychiatry connected with the emotional pains, malaise and aspirations of the populace. The idea of mental health begat images of loving and helping relationships throughout society, even though psychiatry focused largely on the individual.

During the latter half of the century, however, psychiatry lost its soul. We psychiatrists treat mental disorders much more effectively today than we could thirty years ago. We are more honest about the effectiveness of our therapies. Psychiatrists are better medical doctors now, with a greater knowledge of physical science and collaborative working relationships with our medical colleagues. Yet we no longer speak to society's emotional pains. We have learned how to reverse the biological abnormalities that underlie much emotional pain, but we have lost our interest in the care of the soul. Largely due to our better understanding of the brain and a more scientific approach to disordered behavior, we have become brain doctors rather than soul doctors. How did psychiatry lose its soul?

The Flowering of Psychoanalysis in the United States

Psychoanalytically oriented psychiatry infused new life into psychiatry during the 1940s and 1950s, especially in the United States. The new psychiatry spoke to virtually every emotional problem and many physical problems besetting humankind. The public became increasingly aware of psychiatric theories and therapies, they sought psychiatrists as never before, and the United States during the mid-twentieth century was labeled the "psychological society."[2] Not only did psychoanalytically oriented psychiatrists expand their horizons from the problems of everyday life to the most severe psychiatric illnesses (schizophrenia), they also explored the psychological causes of physical illnesses, the mind-body interface.

For example, Franz Alexander explored the mind-body interface through the study of psychosomatic illnesses. He proposed a theory to explain the cause of six chronic physical illnesses: peptic ulcer, asthma, hypertension, rheumatoid arthritis, neurodermatitis and hyperthyroidism.[3] Vectors relating specific psychological conflicts with specific physical illnesses were hypothesized to explain these illnesses. For example, peptic ulcer—erosion of the covering of the upper part of the intestine—develops in the person desiring to be loved and comforted. Milk, which relieves the physical pain of the ulcer, is analogous to mother's milk, which satiates the hungry, loved-starved child. Psychoanalytic therapy was therefore prescribed for relief of these physical illnesses.

The concept of a psychosomatic disorder as proposed by Alexander was philosophically unsound. On the one hand, the concept presupposes a mind-body dualism: the body reflects a conflict parallel to a conflict in the mind. On the other hand, psychoanalysts insisted that physical processes can be reduced to dynamic psychological problems.

René Descartes proposed a similar coexistence for mind and matter as separate realities. Such a view of illness requires that mind and matter interdependently influence each other yet also maintain their status as ontological substances that are, by definition, independent.[4] The mechanistic link between the mind and body was missing and is much more complex than suggested by Alexander. Nevertheless, Alexander's proposed psychosomatic theories were of intuitive appeal to psychiatrists, other physicians and the public. Not only did these theories render psychiatry relevant to the care of the physically ill, they implied that any physician treating these diseases should be grounded in psychiatric as well as physical medicine.

American psychoanalysts also investigated and attempted to treat the devastating disease schizophrenia.[5] Silvano Arieti, Otto Will and Frieda Fromm-Reichmann constructed elaborate theories of the psychological conflicts underlying schizophrenia and developed psychotherapies for this severe disorder. The popular book *I Never Promised You a Rose Garden,*[6] later made into a movie, is the story of Fromm-Reichmann's ongoing psychotherapy with a young schizophrenic woman. These theories maintain that to effectively treat the schizophrenic patient, the psychiatrist must develop a meaningful relationship with him or her. This relationship will theoretically reverse the patient's tendency to withdraw from the environment. Such a relationship will hopefully initiate a new acceptance of reality by the patient, which will then lead the patient to recovery.[7] The popular image of the psychiatrist walking with a troubled patient through the beautiful grounds of a private psychiatric hospital derives from this approach to treating the severely mentally ill. Private psychiatric hospitals such as Shepherd and Enoch Pratt, Highland Hospital, the Institute of Living and the Chestnut Lodge flourished during the 1950s and early 1960s. Patients (who could afford such care) were hospitalized for months, even years, in these pastoral retreats as they slowly struggled to overcome their mental anguish and return to society through the support of caring professionals.

Psychoanalytic therapy was, in some sense, a paradox. On the one hand, the problems that appeared responsive to therapy were individual problems, or intrapsychic problems. Yet the treatment of these problems required a relationship, psychotherapy (albeit a specialized relationship). Care and cure also required withdrawal of the person from society, either during the psychotherapeutic hour or during a hospitalization. Nevertheless, the milieu of the isolated, structured relationship(s) of individual psychotherapy, group psychotherapy or the hospital was central to healing the emotions.

In retrospect, these psychotherapies for both patients with psychosomatic illnesses and those with schizophrenia did not prove cost-effective, and perhaps not effective at all. Today the illnesses previously labeled psycho-somatic illnesses are almost solely medically managed, and supportive psychotherapy is prescribed only for persons experiencing much difficulty in adapting to the illness. Behavioral therapies, such as biofeedback, are prescribed at times, yet these therapies have not been used extensively for the six psychosomatic illnesses of Alexander. Likewise, schizophrenia is treated almost exclusively by medications coupled with behavioral/educational therapies. Therefore we treat these diseases more efficiently and usually more effectively. Therapists are still less apt to consider patients in the context of their ongoing social relations and rarely view the relationship of the doctor to the patient as central to the healing process. Technical expertise is now more valued than interpersonal skills in the doctoring of emotional suffering.

Psychiatry and Society

In 1964 the application of psychiatric theory to the well-being of society was given significant public support in the United States. Dramatically increased funding became available to the National Institute of Mental Health (NIMH), and the passage of the Community Mental Health Act of 1963 mandated NIMH to establish and fund community mental health centers (CMHC) throughout the country. A virtual war on emotional pain was launched, parallel to the more publicized war on poverty. Psychoanalysts and newly emerging social psychiatrists moved away from mainstream medicine and into the community. These social psychiatrists were grounded in the social sciences more than the psychological and biological sciences and emphasized prevention through social intervention rather than individual treatment.

Criticism of institutionalization of the mentally ill in state-supported mental institutions also peaked at this time. Civil rights activists pointed out that many patients had been hospitalized against their will and without evidence that institution-based therapies were beneficial. The physical conditions of the state mental hospitals, in contrast to private facilities, were extremely poor. Staff were untrained, and each psychiatrist was responsible for scores of patients at the same time. New biological therapies, such as the drug Thorazine, helped psychiatrists to control the more severe behavior of schizophrenic patients who required hospitalization.

The advent of the new medications and the CMHC movement accelerated deinstitutionalization, and community mental health centers were expected to meet the needs of these newly discharged, chronically ill patients. Other than medications, however, psychiatry and society were not equipped with proven therapies or systems of care for these patients.[8] We have made tremendous strides in emptying our state mental hospitals, but Americans now live in a society with thousands of homeless individuals, many of whom suffer from severe mental illness and/or substance abuse. The social responsibility felt by psychiatrists working in the early community mental health centers is not paralleled among psychiatrists today. Now psychiatrists working with the homeless focus much more on treating the psychiatric diseases prevalent among them, such as schizophrenia, and less on the social factors contributing to homelessness.

Optimism abounded during the 1960s. Psychiatrists explored new areas, such as family and social interactions, and began to popularize their theories through books, such as Eric Berne's *Games People Play.*[9] Berne loosely adapted Freud's superego (conscience), ego (reality) and id (instinct) to a theory of internalized "parent," "adult" and "child." The parent, adult or child in one person interacts with the parent, adult or child of another, according to Berne. Perhaps one adult initiates what she believes is an adult-to-adult interaction, yet finds she is responded to in a parent-to-child context. These problematic interactions, or the games people play, can be analyzed so that the person can initiate or respond appropriately in future interactions. Berne's easily understood diagnoses and explanations of personal interactions brought Freud's concepts to virtually any reader with a high-school education.

Social psychiatry was most attractive to me during my years of training in psychiatry. Though I was less enthusiastic about the ability of psychosocial theories to change Western society than many of my colleagues, I was convinced that emotional suffering cannot be disowned from its sociocultural context. In other words, relationships are critical to virtually every psychiatric illness and its treatment. Those relationships stretch far beyond the therapist-patient relationship.

Even as psychiatry was spreading its horizons, its foundation as a legitimate medical specialty was eroding from without and from within. From without, a number of events undermined the optimistic views of American society's ability to heal its emotional angst of the 1960s, including the Vietnam War, the outbreak of violence in urban settings, protests on campuses, racial confrontations and the evolution of the drug culture.[10] The hope that the community mental health center movement, undergirded by popularized psychiatric theory, would correct these problems evaporated almost as quickly as it emerged. Psychiatrists withdrew from the community back to hospitals and office practices and became reluctant to provide prescriptions to heal society's ills. America's angst was outside the realm of psychiatry. Psychiatrists returned to treating the more severe psychiatric disorders.

From within, psychiatry was also challenged. Some challenges were frontal, such as psychiatrist Thomas Szasz's suggestion, in *The Myth of Mental Illness,* that many so-called mental illnesses are no more than ordinary problems of living.[11] He suggested, "The notion of a person having a mental illness precludes regarding individuals as responsible persons and invites, instead, treating them as irresponsible patients."[12] The inherent difficulty of differentiating the mentally ill from the worried well was also recognized and utilized by antipsychiatric Christian counselors, who criticized psychiatrists for labeling sin as mental illness (see chapter four).[13]

Michel Foucault, the French philosopher who has been very influential within American universities, extended this critique. He believed that every person's boundaries are restricted by cultural and historical forces that serve institutional rather than individual power. To define normality, a society must isolate certain persons and label them as abnormal. With the rise of capitalism and the Protestant work ethic, the mentally ill could no longer be tolerated as they were in less pressured societies. Therefore the mentally ill had to be labeled and isolated in order to preserve the competitive, individualistic lifestyle of Western society.[14]

I believe Foucault was partially correct. Protestant Christians, especially evangelicals strongly allied with capitalism, did not challenge labeling by psychiatry, despite their criticism of labeling sin as mental illness. They generally supported the individualistic lifestyle; therefore the severely mentally ill were as likely to be segregated from the Christian community as from society as a whole. Despite Foucault's criticism, psychiatry was given responsibility for the medical treatment of the severely mentally ill, but this treatment took place outside the mainstream of society and did not touch society's soul.

Psychiatrist E. Fuller Torey proposed that psychotherapy is little more than a culturally specific healing ritual, similar to that of folk healers in primitive cultures.[15] The scientific foundations of the supposed therapeutic benefit of psychoanalysis and most psychotherapies were questioned. Even the ability of psychoanalysts to distinguish truth from fiction when interpreting the story of a patient was questioned. For example, did the sexual abuse reported by Freud's patients actually represent incidences of sexual abuse or fantasies of the patient?[16] Freud himself questioned the truth of these revelations late in his career, and this debate has flared in recent years as the frequency and severity of child abuse have become more apparent to the public. Rather than aligning itself with the emotionally distressed, psychiatry is often viewed as covering the truth of real abuse with its theories.

These challenges led psychiatrists to question how much they actually did understand their patients. Perhaps we are not nearly as skilled and objective in those so-called therapeutic relationships as we were led to believe when psychoanalysis and social psychiatry were dominant forces. In my own practice I enjoyed learning about the deepest thoughts and feelings of my patients, yet I began to question whether the many hours I spent with some of them was of value. Perhaps Szasz, Foucault and Torey were correct. Perhaps I brought erroneous preconceived views to some of the relationships and doomed them from the beginning.

Psychiatry also began to experience internal competition for increasingly scarce resources during the early 1970s. The payers for mental health services visualized psychiatry and psychoanalysis as bottomless pits requiring unlimited resources.[17] As the bottom line emerged as a dominant theme in the delivery of health care, those who sought to contain costs scrutinized psychiatric services. Simultaneously, Christian counselors and counselors from a vast array of other theoretical orientations were growing in number. Armed with degrees in psychology, social work, and marriage and family therapy, they were positioned to compete directly with psychiatrists for Christian clients desiring mental health services.

Psychiatry thus entered the 1970s in a state of uncertainty and restlessness, finding it difficult to abandon its psychoanalytic roots yet uncomfortably isolated from other medical specialties. Psychiatry had clearly failed in its goal to improve community mental health through social action. From this uncertainty and crisis in identity, neuropsychiatry emerged to dominate psychiatry within a decade.

Neuropsychiatry, as a category within psychiatry, became the means for psychiatrists to emphasize their focus on the biological as opposed to psychoanalytic and social psychiatry. The foundations of a biological psychiatry date from antiquity, though it was overshadowed by psychoanalysis from the 1920s to the 1960s. Throughout this period neuropsychiatry was not dead but was quietly developing its own models of psychopathology and biological therapies. Many biologically oriented psychiatrists had long awaited the opportunity to recapture the field they had lost to Freud and the community mental health center movement. As in the nineteenth century, neuropsychiatrists had little interest in religion in general and Christianity in particular as they related to psychiatric disorders. They had virtually no concern about the neurotic basis of religion and therefore no desire to converse with or debate Christian theologians and counselors. They had little desire to prescribe cures for society's ills but wished to become respected medical specialists treating persons with specific psychiatric disorders.

The Rise of Psychopharmacology

Psychiatric therapy has ancient roots in biology. Hippocrates, four centuries before the Christian era, criticized Greek superstition regarding epilepsy, the "sacred disease." He stated: "Men ought to know that from nothing else but thence [from the brain] comes joys, delights, laughter in sports and sorrows, griefs, despondency and lamentations . . . and by the same organ we become mad and delirious."[18]

Biological therapies and isolation continued to dominate the treatment of severe emotional illness until the emergence of Freud. Treatments such as cathartics and physical exercise were prominent during the Middle Ages. At the beginning of the twentieth century, therapies such as vitamins to address dietary deficiencies (mental problems resulting from pellagra, for example, are caused by a deficiency in nicotinic acid) and medications such as chloral hydrate, a potent sedative, were widely used. Even during the days of the rapid growth of psychoanalysis, biological therapies were being discovered and perfected. Ugo Cerletti and Lucio Beni introduced electro-convulsive treatments (ECT, or electroshock) as a therapy for a variety of severe mental disorders in 1938.

Yet the emergence of neuropsychiatry as the dominant paradigm for investigating and treating mental disorders in America derived from the psychopharmacological revolution of the late 1950s and 1960s. During a fifteen-year period, from about 1950 to 1965, four medications were introduced which increased the efficacy of psychiatric treatment tremendously. The derivatives of these medications are still the mainstays of psychophar-macological therapy of mental illness.

Thorazine, an antipsychotic drug, was introduced during the early 1950s and was the first drug to effectively control the symptoms of schizophrenia. Thorazine and its descendants, such as Haldol and Clozaril, were the most important contributors to the dramatic decline in the census of mental hospitals from the early 1950s until today.

Tofranil was introduced during the late 1950s and is the progenitor of all antidepressant medications such as Elavil and Prozac. It reduced the need for electroshock therapy and effectively treated the episodic severe depressions of persons who had not responded to psychotherapy.

Librium, an antianxiety drug, was first used in 1960 and was the proto-type of the frequently prescribed drugs Valium and Xanax. During the mid-1960s, lithium, a naturally occurring salt, was successfully used in controlling the mood swings of manic-depressive patients. Thorazine, Tofranil, Librium and lithium were proven effective in carefully performed scientific studies. The range of disorders they treated, from schizophrenia to anxiety, included most of the more severe problems psychiatrists treat.

Unlike psychoanalysis, neuropsychiatric theory followed neuropsychiatric practice. The serendipitous success of these four psychotropic medications led to the emergence of theories of mental illness based on brain pathology. During the 1960s neuropsychiatrists posited that "chemical imbalances," with the chemicals varying by illness, could be responsible for illnesses. For example, the chemical messenger dopamine was postulated to be out of balance in schizophrenia. Norepinephrine and serotonin were among the chemical messengers postulated to be out of balance in depression and manic-depressive illness.

These theories of chemical imbalance initially derived from the known effects of medications on brain function coupled with the known effect of medications on psychiatric symptoms. For example, Tofranil increases the concentration of the neurotransmitter norepinephrine in the gap between two nerve cells. These chemical messengers facilitate or inhibit transfer of electrical impulses from one nerve cell to another. Depression was postulated to be caused by a decreased concentration of norepinephrine within nerve cells in certain parts of the brain. Psychiatrists therefore began to see depression as analogous to the way an internist sees diabetes—as the result of a chemical imbalance in the production of insulin.

We now know that the biological basis of depression is more complex, involving not only levels of neurotransmitters but also regulating sites for binding these transmitters. Still, the emergence during the 1960s of theories explaining psychiatric illness as a chemical imbalance set the stage for the ascendance of a brain-based psychiatry. Neuropsychiatrists had no more need to consider the social, cultural and religious in the diagnosis and treatment of a psychiatric illness than did the internist in the treatment of diabetes.

The history of psychiatry in America during the later twentieth century is the history of the ascendance of neuropsychiatry. Neuropsychiatry is not a new phenomenon, for Emil Kraeplin in Europe and his predecessors during the nineteenth century were most interested in the brain and the phenomena of behavior that result from brain pathology (see chapter one). Tools available to the psychiatrist in recent years, however, have permitted visualization and quantification of brain function in ways that were unheard-of twenty years ago. Not only can concentrations of chemical messengers be measured in the blood and the fluid that bathes the brain (cerebral spinal fluid), but the sites where these messengers attach to nerve cells can be studied directly in the brains of animals and humans.

Most views of the function of the brain are through the window of chemical messengers and their receptors on the nerve cells. This is the study of the means by which the brain transmits an impulse from one nerve cell to the next. The location of various types of receptors throughout the brain, the activity of these receptors in the presence of radioactively labeled chemical messengers and the behavioral consequences of stimulating or blocking normal messenger function are at the heart of modern neuroscience and neuropsychiatry. In other words, mind has been reduced to brain, and brain has been reduced in large part to neural networks, much like a microchip.

Neuropsychiatrists do recognize more complex integrative activities of the brain which occur beyond simple messenger-receptor activity (such as neural networks). But because these integrative activities are most difficult to study, they are relegated to the back burner of neuropsychiatric exploration. The search for simple mechanisms predominates. In contrast, interest in integrative mechanisms has become a major focus among experimental neuroscientists. Recent books written for the general public by established neuroscientists, including *The Engine of Reason, the Seat of the Soul* by Paul Churchland and *Consciousness Explained* by Daniel Dennett, propose bold theories of the basis of mind, soul and even religious sentiment.[19]

One consequence of the rise of neuropsychiatry has been a paradigm shift from verbal to visual in the approach to psychiatric investigation. This shift follows the societal trend toward an almost unquenchable desire for images. When I browse through the pages of the *American Journal of Psychiatry* from the 1950s and 1960s, I occasionally find a table and only rarely a photograph. A review of the journal in 1995 reveals tables and figures in virtually every article, and photographs or diagrams in many. These photographs result from new and powerful techniques for visualizing the brain, including magnetic resonance imaging (MRI) and positron emission tomography (PET). Verbal description is less valued as information relevant to diagnosis and treatment of emotional problems than information that can be diagrammed, quantified and imaged. This visual information is typically frozen in time, a snapshot rather than a motion picture.

The paradigm for understanding psychiatric disorders has likewise shifted from the process of hearing a patient's complaints unfold through time to the snapshot diagnostic interview and diagnostic test. The story of the psychiatric patient is therefore less valued. "A picture is worth a thousand words" is as true for modern psychiatry as it is for the treatment of cancer of the liver, despite the fact that virtually no psychiatric illness can be identified by an imaging technique.

Psychiatry is not unusual in its pursuit of the visual; our society has welcomed the image. Typical television commercials are brief images, often only fifteen to thirty seconds long, not carefully arranged arguments for buying one product versus another. Though the mind functions as a stream of consciousness through time and is capable of full expression only by narrative, the unfolding of concepts appears to have diminishing relevance to both the psychiatrist and society as a whole. If the psychiatrist can "see" an chemical abnormality in the blood or an abnormal image on an MRI and can verify that the abnormality has been corrected visually, such as in the normalization of the lab value, then the practice of psychiatry can, in theory, be effected by discrete, limited contacts with the patient. Ongoing verbal interaction between psychiatrist and patient, the therapeutic relationship, is perceived as less important. Soul talk, sharing the deepest of thoughts and fears and being understood by a doctor of the soul, has faded dramatically as an expectation by the psychiatric patient.

Even as the discovery of the antidepressant Tofranil helped stimulate the reemergence of neuropsychiatry, the study of the brain and its specific messengers and receptors has stimulated the development of new and more specific neuropsychiatric medications. Prozac and its relatives Zoloft, Paxil and Serzone belong to a family of drugs called the selective serotonin reuptake inhibitors (SSRIs). Compared to older antidepressants, such as Tofranil and Elavil, these drugs work more specifically on the serotonin messenger system. While they are no more effective overall than the older antidepressants, they do produce fewer side effects.

Concurrent with the marketing of these drugs, however, new biologic theories of personality have emerged, connecting specific personality types with specific chemical messengers, especially serotonin, norepinephrine and dopamine. Personality types, the introvert for example, are theorized to result from the balance of activity across these chemical messengers. Medications can theoretically change the basic personality of those taking them by readjusting the levels of these messengers. Psychiatrists have reported that Prozac does appear to change personality in some patients. Depressed patients who respond to Tofranil might say after successful treatment, "I think I am back to normal." Patients taking Prozac, however, at times say, "I have never been so outgoing in my life. Wow! This is great stuff." Just such responses led Peter Kramer to write his popular book *Listening to Prozac*.[20]

The response of society to Prozac has been quite different from its response during the 1960s to the early antidepressants. People speak not only of antidepressant or antianxiety drugs but also of designer drugs, that is, "made-to-order, off-the-shelf" personalities and moods.[21] With medications emerging to alter or redirect personality and mood, a reductionistic psychobiology of religion cannot be far behind. Yet psychiatrists, pastoral counselors and theologians have been virtually unaware of, uncritical of and unconcerned about this revolution in psychiatry and have embraced neuropsychiatry with open arms.

Critique and concern by psychiatrists of neuropsychiatry should not be based in a desire for people to suffer when relief is available, but rather based on the trend toward blind acceptance of relief from a pill. Many committed Christians with no serious mental disorders have sought my services specifically for a prescription of Prozac. Christian counselors and pastors have quickly deferred to me when emotional pain persists, and Christian patients referred to me have willingly accepted almost every drug prescribed. Though some Christians continue to resist medications, the trend is clearly toward acceptance.

Psychiatrists should take the lead in expressing caution about solving emotional angst by taking a pill. Doctors of the soul will distinguish between the proper use of medication for treating psychiatric disorders and the inappropriate desire to cure social and existential pain with a pill.

The Psychopharmacology of Religion

Suggestions that personality and even spiritual sentiments are biological phenomena are not unique to psychiatrists of the late twentieth century. Hippocrates postulated that temperament is based on the relative balance of four body "humors": blood for sanguine, designating warmth, cheerfulness and optimism; black bile for melancholic, a tendency toward sadness or depression; yellow bile for choleric, designating anger; and phlegm for phlegmatic, designating sluggishness and apathy.[22] Robert Burton (seventeenth century), who was convinced that his melancholy derived from the pressures of the devil and the priest, recommended that "the best means to reduce them [religious melancholic feelings] to a sound mind is to alter their course of life with constant threats, promises, persuasions, and intermixed physick."[23] "Physick" for Burton was medication, diet, bathing, moderate exercise, reading, clean air and travel abroad, all intended to correct the balance of the humors.

G. Stanley Hall, a nineteenth-century psychologist, observed that most conversion experiences occur around the time of puberty, parallel to the physical changes accompanying sexual maturation. He suggested that religious devotion and sexual love share many similarities, such as tendencies to vacillate between self-assertion and self-abnegation, to become overly dedicated to objects of devotion, to express devotion in rhythmic music and dance, and to feel ecstatically and invincibly happy.[24] Hall's psychological theories were based on Hippocratic ideas about temperament. In his view, religious sentiment is in no way dependent on a transcendent Other. In Hall's autobiography he reflects that "every item of my psychology and philosophy, whether acquired or original, grew out of my . . . basal and instinctual traits."[25]

The study of the biology of religion reemerged in America during the 1950s and 1960s, with advances in neuropsychiatry. Arnold Mandell postulated in 1978 that transcendental experience can be explored through modern neurochemical, neuropharmacological and neurophysiological techniques.[26] He argued that mood disturbances in persons with manic-depressive illness, the ecstasies accompanying epileptic seizures, the transcendent consciousness induced by hallucinogenic drugs and meditation all represent similar neurobiological phenomena. These phenomena begin with loss of normal inhibition caused by an imbalance of serotonin in the temporal lobe of the brain. Such imbalances lead to increased brain discharges, which result in phenomena ranging from pleasure to ecstasy. Diverse experiences can emerge from such neurobiological mechanisms. A shift from fear and hate to virtual idolatrous love for their captors among some hijacking victims (the so-called Stockholm effect), the brainwashing of persons to an entirely new philosophical and emotional state, the ecstatic experience of the long-distance runner, and the creative moment following hours and days of intellectual struggle are among these experiences.[27] Biological mechanisms, Mandell argued, undergird even the transcendent experience of God.

This philosophy of human nature, a neurobiologic explanation of the religious impulse, is also expounded by many biologists from other disciplines as well as psychiatrists and neuroscientists. Edward O. Wilson, the Pulitzer prize-winning world authority on ants, sums up this philosophy:

> Religion itself is subject to the explanations of the natural sciences. . . . Psychobiology can account for the very origin of mythology [religion] by the principle of natural selection acting on the genetically evolved material structure of the human brain. . . . The final decisive edge enjoyed by scientific naturalism will come from its capacity to explain traditional religion, its chief competitor, as a wholly material phenomena. Theology is not likely to survive as an independent intellectual discipline.[28]

Not all biologists and neuropsychiatrists are so reductionistic. For example, well-known evolutionary biologist Ernst Mayr does not believe "definite genes controlling character traits of high ethical value have ever been demonstrated."[29] Though Mayr does not postulate a transcendent God, he does accept an individual's "capacity for adopting ethical behavior beyond genes and molecules."[30] He leaves room for something beyond heredity, namely, the interaction of genetic programs for development with the environment.

Neuropsychiatrists, however, have scarcely considered the philosophical, much less the theological, implications of their scientific explorations. I found it therefore most refreshing to read the works of my friend and colleague Ed Hundert from Harvard. In his *Philosophy, Psychiatry and Neuroscience: A Synthetic Analysis of the Varieties of Human Experience,* he takes great care not to overextend the reaches of a synthesis of psychology and brain biology, even within a firmly grounded philosophical framework.[31] He carefully separates the metaphysical mind-body question (and for our purposes the problem of a transcendent God and the ability of humankind to know that God) from the epistemological problems. Hundert recognizes that the metaphysical question "What actually exists?" cannot be addressed by a study of psychology and neuroscience based in traditional philosophy. But the epistemological problem "How is it possible to realize valid knowledge?" can be addressed.

Even addressing this problem must avoid the illusion of a totally objective brain (or brain science). Hundert incorporates the honest concept "intersubjectivity" to frame explanations of both normal behavior and emotional suffering. In the last analysis, Hundert basically affirms that we can never be absolutely objective as individuals. Interrelationships provide checks and balances on our subjective analyses. If we accept interrelations with a spiritual being, God, then we can know, though not perfectly, that which is beyond the physical, the metaphysical.

Unfortunately, the works of Mayr and Hundert are scarcely considered as neuropsychiatrists plow forward to discover the biological seat of emotional suffering devoid of relations. Arnold Cooper, in evaluating the impact of neuropsychiatry, suggests that neurophysiological advances will continue the centuries-old attempt to confine the realm of the psyche, but there is no danger that mind will disappear. For instance, years ago even tuberculosis was considered primarily a mental illness. Then the tubercular bacillus was identified as the ultimate causative agent. Even so, many persons who are host to the bacillus never develop the disease; many factors, especially the relation of the host to the social environment, contribute to the onset of the disease. The chemical imbalances underlying the most severe depressions are today recognized by virtually all physicians as well as the lay public. Nevertheless, according to Cooper, neurobiology will never be the bridge to the unconscious, for neurobiology explains at a different level from psychology.

Cooper believes that knowledge of the brain should not fundamentally alter our mode of inquiring about the mind.[32] I agree with him (he is a good friend with whom I have discussed these issues in some depth). We cannot return to the dualism of Descartes, yet a completely materialistic approach to consciousness, the unconscious and especially self-consciousness is difficult to defend.

One approach that retains the knowledge of biological mechanisms yet does not assume a reductionistic approach is *supervenience*. Properties of one kind, such as consciousness, supervene on properties of another kind, such as neurochemical transmission of an impulse from one nerve cell to another. The underlying property must be there, but the supervening property cannot be deduced to the underlying property. Therefore different avenues of inquiry into the thoughts and behavior of humankind are necessary if we are to avoid the deterministic, and frankly, depressing limits of a purely materialistic approach.

Even if mechanistic neuropsychiatry is philosophically unsound, however, its influence is pervasive. Melvin Sabshin sums up the influence of neuropsychiatry as follows. "The borders and boundaries of psychiatry that seemed infinite in the 1960s became somewhat narrower. . . . By 1989, our field is dominated by a remedicalization, a predominance of science over ideology, and a tendency toward boundary circumspection."[33]

If religious experience can be reduced to specific neurobiological mechanisms, such as alterations of the serotonin system of chemical messengers, then medications that affect these chemical messengers could alter religious as well as personal experiences.

Peter Kramer, in *Listening to Prozac*,[34] does not focus on the new generation of antidepressants for their ability to relieve the severely depressed, but rather for their potential to alter personality. Prozac affects the chemical messenger serotonin, which Mandell associates with religious experiences. Though Kramer does not address religion directly, he comes close to suggesting that the ethical and religious values of an individual can be altered by medications if they are obstacles to full self-realization. "Psychotherapeutic medication . . . leads us to focus on biological differences, . . . to the extent that medications are an important agent for personal transformation."[35] In other words, personality and temperament can be understood and changed by the new antidepressants, though these changes were previously reserved for learning through relationship psychotherapy (where results were questionable) and religion, especially religious conversion (a change in relationship with the person's perception of a transcendent Other).

What are the ethical implications of using Prozac as a drug to alter personality and perhaps one's worldview as well? I believe they are profound.

Kramer emphasizes yet another critical issue associated with neuropsychiatry, namely, its application to the populace as well as the psychiatric patient: "In time, I suspect we will come to discover that modern psychopharmacology has become, like Freud in his day, a whole climate of opinion under which we conduct our different lives."[36] Drugs such as Prozac and Valium are not only accepted but embedded in our culture. Persons, both Christian and non-Christian, now ask for Prozac rather than expressing pain, dysfunction or even mild dissatisfaction with themselves. They don't seek help with their relations with others and with God but rather seek to feel better, assuming that the relations will improve if they feel better.

Psychiatrists, even those embedded in strong faith traditions, either have ignored or are unaware of society's response to the perceived effects of these designer drugs. Simple responses such as "God has provided these medications, and we should thank him for making them available" or "Christians should not use mind-altering drugs" are not sufficient. Antidepressant medications are safe, are not addictive and can bring relief to thousands of persons suffering the severe symptoms of depression. Yet should a medication be the first solution considered when a person feels emotional pain?[37] The implicit message from psychiatrists and other physicians who prescribe these drugs indiscriminately is that unhappiness is biological and can be cured with a pill.

The physician is (or should be) trained to understand the cause of a person's suffering, and if that cause is, for example, disordered relations or a sick culture, then a drug is not the solution. During a busy day in the life of the practicing physician, however, it is all too easy to prescribe a drug rather than sort out a complicated psychosocial (and perhaps spiritual) problem described by the patient. Most busy doctors spend less than five minutes discussing an emotional problem with a patient. Patients, in turn, are quick to accept medications because they expect their doctor to do something and they wish the answer to their problems to be as simple as a pill. Yet many of the most meaningful religious experiences arise from emotional suffering that persists over weeks and months, suffering that does not lend itself to easy answers.

The danger of neuropsychiatry to religion, however, must not be over-stated. Mandell wrote of specific religious experiences as opposed to general religious behavior when he proposed a biological basis for religion. Psychoactive drugs are even used to produce experiences that are believed to be spiritual. Native Americans use peyote, a psychedelic drug, as a central element in their religious practices to relate to the spiritual world. Though this practice rarely leads to drug abuse or dysfunctional behavior, society as a whole has taken a negative view of the practice. Native Americans are at times punished under state antidrug regulations for their religious prac-tices. Likewise, there are many persons in our society wary of Prozac. Psychiatrists in the United Kingdom have commented to me that the British are typically reticent to use antidepressant drugs, and many general practi-tioners are reticent to prescribe them. Prozac use is sometimes considered analogous to abuse of illicit drugs. Western society has not accepted drugs unequivocally as the answer to its problems.

Nevertheless, the trend is clearly toward more widespread use and uncritical acceptance of psychopharmacology in the United States, and therefore caution is in order, especially from those psychiatrists interested in the person as well as a specific psychiatric symptom. In the closing pages of Aldous Huxley's *Brave New World,* a group of reporters have difficulty understanding the reality of pain felt by "the savage." They shout, "Why don't you take Soma? . . . Evil's an unreality if you take a couple of grams. . . . Pain's a delusion."[38] When Huxley wrote these words in 1932, few of his readers could imagine that humankind would become so fearful of feeling pain that they would accept medicine to relieve pain without questioning its use.

Pain is a necessity, and people can lose their identity and the ability to protect themselves if they do not experience pain. We have moved toward Huxley's "brave new world" during the past quarter century as we drugged emotional pain and suffering with our own forms of Soma. Uncritical acceptance of neuropsychiatry implies a step toward the dystopia of Huxley. Psychiatrists have been all too indifferent to the new prescription-drug culture, even as they battle the use of street drugs. How have psychiatrists lost sight of the larger picture? Specialization and medicalization of psychiatry take much of the soul from psychiatry.

The Specialization and Medicalization of Psychiatry

Medicine has increasingly become specialized during the past twenty-five years. The overspecialization of American physicians became a central topic during the health care reform debate in the mid 1990s. State and federal governments are pushing for a shift toward generalists or primary care physicians because they are anticipated to be the gatekeepers of health services, the physicians who treat the whole person, in the future. The public, however, may not be aware of the main reason for specialization in American medicine. Most assume it is simply a desire for increased financial security and status, but these desires are only a part of the reason that American physicians have moved toward specialization. The explosion of medical science and the technological sophistication of diagnostic procedures, coupled with the emergence of more complicated therapies, has left many physicians feeling unqualified to practice across disciplines. In other words, they don't feel comfortable dealing with the whole person, body and soul. Only by specializing can physicians feel competent, having truly mastered an area of medical practice.

Psychiatry, like other medical disciplines, moved toward increased specialization during the 1970s with the emergence of subspecialties including psychopharmacology, geriatric psychiatry, forensic psychiatry and addiction psychiatry. Prior to the 1970s, the only important subspecialty of psychiatry was child psychiatry. The reasons for psychiatry's specialization during the 1970s were the same as for the other medical specialties. Psychiatrists felt more comfortable when they knew almost everything about one area of psychiatry rather than a little about all areas. I felt this push to specialize early in my career and therefore focused on the psychiatry of old age (geriatric psychiatry) and the empirical study of psychiatric disorders in the community (psychiatric epidemiology). I even went so far as to obtain a Ph.D. in epidemiology.

Yet "specialization" implies the use of special tools and techniques. Before 1970 there was little use of the laboratory in psychiatry. Over the past twenty-five years, however, the laboratory tests available to the psychiatrist have increased dramatically, including improved methods for viewing brain structure (MRI) and brain function (PET). In addition, a long-used diagnostic procedure for epilepsy, the electroencephalogram (EEG), has been quantified and submitted to computer analysis, producing "pictures" of the brain derived from these tracings of brain electrical activity.

It remains unclear to what extent these diagnostic tests have improved the care of psychiatric patients, since the likelihood of identifying previously unknown treatable problems via these testing procedures is low and the tests rarely inform the approach to therapy. They are of great value, however, in the exploration of brain structure and function among persons with and without psychiatric disorders. Laboratory diagnostic tests have been widely used in recent years by psychiatrists.

Why have these tests become so attractive to psychiatrists? For one, they permit psychiatrists to actually *see* the brain, both its structure and its function. These pictures of the brain are constructed from numerical data rather than actual photographs, and they are subject to considerable misinterpretation. Despite this, by using these tests psychiatrists have joined other medical specialists in viewing the problems of their patients directly. Just as the gastroenterologist can, by using a gastroscope, view the lining of the stomach and diagnose a gastric ulcer, the psychiatrist can view an MRI scan and confirm the diagnosis of Huntington's disease. Additionally, anatomical brain changes have been found to be associated with certain psychiatric illnesses. For example, the ventricles—cavities in the center of the brain that contain cerebral spinal fluid—tend to be enlarged in schizophrenia. The diagnostic and therapeutic value of these changes has yet to be established.

Psychiatrists also examine blood samples. Though none of the common psychiatric disorders can be diagnosed by a blood test, some chemical abnormalities are associated with psychiatric symptoms, such as depression and anxiety. For example, the dexamethasone suppression test (DST) has been used for years to diagnose Cushing's disease, in which the body produces abnormally high levels of cortisol because of an overactive adrenal gland. Cortisol is a hormone that is secreted into the bloodstream at times of stress. Persons experiencing depression produce more cortisol than normal, perhaps because severe depression is stressful to the body. Psychiatrists using the DST have demonstrated an association between high levels of cortisol production and severe depression. The DST has therefore been used as a diagnostic test for depression.

In reality, the DST provides the psychiatrist with limited useful information beyond what can be learned by talking with the patient. Rarely are treatment decisions based on results of the DST. The test is of some value in predicting the efficacy of certain treatments. If a depressed patient is given an antidepressant medication following an abnormal DST but does not appear to improve after a couple of weeks, the psychiatrist may repeat the DST. If the cortisol level has dropped, chances are the depression will improve over the next couple of weeks. The body's chemistry appears to reflect the recovery before the person experiences the recovery. This test has been used most often by psychiatrists, however, as a biological marker of depression—that is, an abnormal test marks or identifies a severe depression. Even though this marker is not necessary for diagnostic decisions, psychiatrists feel more comfortable when they can mimic other physicians by using laboratory tests as diagnostic aids.

Paradoxically, other medical specialties are now questioning the widespread use of laboratory tests, because they are expensive and in many cases not proven useful. For example, the value of PSA (prostatic-specific antigen) as a screening test for prostate cancer is questionable in men over the age of seventy, though it is widely used at present.

Armed with these new diagnostic procedures and medications, psychiatrists practice their specialty in a manner similar to the internist, the neurologist and the family physician. A brief history and physical examination are followed by laboratory tests, which in turn are followed by the prescription of a drug or other therapy. This pattern of practice is comfortable to psychiatrists who do not wish to lose their identity as physicians. No doubt effective tests will emerge to better diagnose the more severe psychiatric disorders in the future. Yet the general practice of psychiatry should never be dominated by laboratory tests. Most common emotional problems are best identified by listening to patients. Listening is the soul of good diagnostic medicine; it is through listening that the fractured relations of those who are emotionally suffering are revealed.

Though psychiatrists in the past were loath to wear white coats and practiced for the most part in offices or in psychiatric hospitals separated from general hospitals, they now have returned to the white coat and general hospital. When I leave my office, I always put on my white coat and am even tempted to carry a stethoscope. Psychiatrists may see as many as twenty-five patients a day for fifteen to thirty minutes each. During an afternoon of practice I typically see ten patients, whereas in the past a full day's practice consisted of seeing seven patients for an hour each. General psychiatric clinics have been replaced by specialty clinics, such as eating disorder clinics, mood disorder clinics, anxiety and panic disorder clinics, phobic disorder clinics, and attention deficit disorder clinics.

The investigation and treatment of patients with similar symptoms in specialty clinics has facilitated the collection of vast amounts of empirical information about these patients. Thirty years ago, a clinical investigator could easily publish her or his findings on a series of six patients with, for example, anorexia nervosa, suggesting that experience with these six patients could be generalized to much broader categories. Today an acceptable clinical study must include scores of patients analyzed with appropriate statistical tests. These larger studies have helped psychiatrists be less hasty in accepting new forms of therapy or associating a psychiatric disorder with a particular cause. Yet the individual case report of unique characteristics of patients, the patient's story, is now deemed less useful for improving psychiatric practice than in the past. What we gain in accuracy from the larger studies we lose in not encountering each patient as a special person in relation with others and with spiritual longings.

The general psychiatrist is now less capable of keeping current with clinically relevant research, especially research into treatment with medications. Subspecialties naturally resulted. Psychopharmacology was among the first subspecialties to establish themselves within psychiatry. The challenges of prescribing drugs for psychiatric disorders have been complicated enough to justify additional training, and it soon became clear that gaining extensive experience in psychopharmacology might mean a psychiatrist could not also acquire skills in psychotherapy. Other areas of special expertise have subsequently emerged. For example, psychiatric care of older adults is a complex endeavor, so some psychiatrists now seek specialized fellowship training in geriatric psychiatry. The American Board of Psychiatry and Neurology offers a certificate of "added qualification" in geriatric psychiatry for psychiatrists who complete fellowship training and pass a written examination. I am so certified and, in fact, have made my academic and clinical reputation in large part as a geriatric psychiatrist specializing in the study and treatment of depression in late life.

How have the medicalization and specialization of psychiatry affected the conversation between psychiatry and Christianity? First, psychiatrists have been much less concerned with comprehensive theories of the causes of emotional suffering, which include biological, psychological, social and spiritual factors. This result of specialization has been described by José Ortega y Gasset.[39] Ortega perhaps overstates the case, but he suggests that specialists in politics, art or the sciences are primitive and ignorant, yet perceive themselves as self-sufficient. They are self-satisfied within their limitations and have little ability to resist the flow of a society in matters outside their perceived areas of specialization. Ortega goes further:

> If the specialist is ignorant of the entire philosophy of the science he cultivates, he is much more radically ignorant of the historical conditions requisite for its continuation; that is to say: how society and the heart of man are to be organized in order that they may continue to be investigators.[40]

The specialist in psychiatry has less interest in the larger issues that stimulated Freud, Menninger, Jung and other psychiatrists in the early and mid-twentieth century. Psychiatrists have lost interest in sociology, anthro-

pology, philosophy and theology in general, and specifically have lost
interest in the philosophy of the sciences that undergird the practice of
modern psychiatry. Medicalization and specialization in psychiatry *is* undergirded by a philosophy, and one aspect of that philosophy is a radical
medical empiricism. Operational psychiatry is the consequence of this
empiricism.

Operational Psychiatry

As psychiatrists developed specialized biological explanations and interventions for virtually all human experiences, they abandoned interest in the
personal meaning of emotional pain and suffering to their patients. To
facilitate the prescription of neuropsychiatric therapies, it was perceived
more important to describe than to explain. The rich, though perhaps
distorted, psychological and social explanations of psychiatric disorders
developed by Freud and elaborated by his followers have given way to a
descriptive psychiatry focused on symptoms and behaviors that can be
observed and measured. All medical practitioners feel compelled to name
or label a problem before they can cure it, just as the young woman in the
fairy tale was compelled to name Rumpelstiltskin before she could gain
power over him.

The desire to label has not changed during my career, but the approach
to labeling has changed. Descriptive psychiatry in the United States culminated in the publication of the third edition of the *Diagnostic and Statistical
Manual of Mental Disorders* (DSM-III).[41] The *Diagnostic and Statistical
Manual,* since it was first published in 1952, has been the bible for labeling
in psychiatry. DSM-III was a radical departure from previous diagnostic
manuals in American psychiatry. DSM-III and its successors, DSM-IIIR
(1987) and DSM-IV (1994), virtually abandoned previous attempts by
psychiatrists to include explanations of causation within the labels they
used. The new classifications are instead based on reliable observation.[42]

For example, in earlier DSM editions, depression was defined in large
part based on its presumed cause. Involutional melancholia was a severe
depression *caused by* the involutional period of a woman's biological
development, or menopause. With time psychiatrists recognized that evi-

dence for a depression specifically caused by menopause was virtually nonexistent. Many other time-honored explanations of psychiatric disorders evaporated, leading to a profound skepticism among psychiatrists about our ability to identify specific causes of psychiatric disorders. We therefore adopted a descriptive, empirical approach to diagnosis. Major depression was defined in DSM-III not by its cause but by the presence or absence of certain symptoms such as sleep disturbance, decreased appetite and suicidal thoughts. The test this new approach must pass is the reliability of the diagnosis, whether two or more psychiatrists can agree on the diagnosis after each has talked with and examined the patient.

The reliability of a diagnosis is a measure of the extent to which clinicians who independently observe a person suffering an emotional problem can agree on what to label the problem. Reliability can be increased when the criteria for diagnoses are *operational.* The operational approach to diagnosis derives from the operational theory of the physicist Percy Bridgman.[43] Operationalism defines scientific contents in terms of the actual experimental procedures or operations used to establish their applicability. For example, length is defined by the operations by which it is measured, such as the use of a measuring rod. The physicist therefore should not debate the "true" length of a meter but should accept a particular rod as the standard. A meter is the length of a particular rod. Likewise, major depression is defined in DSM-IV by the accumulation of five or more observable symptoms that can be reliably recorded by a psychiatrist during a diagnostic interview.

Operationalism is a radically empiricist approach to science. I find this new approach to labeling more honest and predictable. When I label a person with major depression, I have limited my own biases and can feel reasonable certainty that a colleague will assign the same label to this patient. Yet the labels have a tendency to take on a life of their own. The label somehow becomes "truth," as it represents an actual and singular condition. Nevertheless, the people I label with "major depression" come in a variety of forms and, it seems to me, range from persons with severe biological illness to persons experiencing a transient mood change, perhaps secondary to chronic stress in the workplace. Psychiatrists who are interested in the classification of emotional suffering focus on recognizing symptoms rather than searching for the cause of those symptoms, since cause must be inferred. Discovering or interpreting the meaning of an emotional problem to a patient is not the goal. Classifying the patient becomes the goal. Why?

Operational, reliable diagnoses render the assignment of specific therapies much easier. Just as measuring a blood pressure of 180/100 in a young woman leads almost automatically to the prescription of an antihypertensive drug, assigning an operational diagnosis of major depression of moderate severity to a middle-aged man leads to the prescription of an antidepressant drug. In a busy office practice, once I have assigned a label I am not obligated to explore in depth the context of the emotional suffering. Even if I prescribe psychotherapy, the therapy is tailored not so much to the specific problems of this middle-aged man as to the generic problem "major depression." Operational diagnoses are simple but sterile.

I emphasize that operational psychiatry is a more honest psychiatry. Psychiatrists during the early and mid-twentieth century were biased observers. One psychiatrist would assume that a woman was suffering from a severe depression based on conflicts experienced with her mother. Another would assume the same woman was anxious (not depressed) because of a difficult adjustment to a work situation. These two psychiatrists would view the same phenomenon but would label it differently based on their theoretical orientations. The operational approach does not seek an explanation of the symptoms. Rather, the psychiatrist observes and records the symptoms. Once these symptoms are cataloged, they are applied to an algorithm to determine the diagnosis. Psychiatrists using the operational approach are very reliable, although the operational approach does not consider the spiritual and the existential aspects of emotional suffering. It deemphasizes the social aspects. The spiritual, social and existential do not lend themselves to easy agreement between psychiatrists and therefore muddy an otherwise relatively clear approach to labeling.

The impact of the operational approach on psychiatric practice has been as profound as the impact of advances in neurobiology. Psychiatry, for the most part, has abandoned the exploration of each emotional problem as a unique problem for which a unique psychological and social explanation should be discovered. Modern psychiatrists fit their patients into the Procrustean bed of the diagnostic categories of the DSM system. The psychiatrist at midcentury was at times guilty of trying to fit diverse symptoms to a common cause such as sexual inhibitions, but the modern psychiatrist has been at least as guilty of overconcern with "goodness of fit." Individuality and the unique life story of the patient, central to psychiatric practice at midcentury, have become peripheral to diagnosis and treatment. Patients are square or round pegs to be fitted into their respective holes. If the peg doesn't fit due to problems of soul, the person is often ignored. The patient, of course, does not understand her or his emotional problem as an entity based on a cluster of symptoms. Emotional suffering is a personal experience and is unique to the life events, values, sentiments and relationships of the individual.

The DSM system does acknowledge the spiritual. A new diagnostic code has been introduced in DSM-IV to designate psychoreligious or psychospiritual problems. Examples of such problems include questioning of a firmly held faith or difficulty following conversion to a new faith.[44] Other examples are near-death experiences and mystical experiences. Some welcome this addition as an accommodation between psychiatry and religion, a more culturally sensitive diagnostic system.[45] Unfortunately, in this accommodation religion itself becomes operationalized; religious experiences are relegated to observable and measurable phenomena. Religious phenomena are viewed as either risk or supportive factors that modify the actual phenomenon of interest—the psychiatric symptom.

Recent investigations of the interface between psychiatry and religion from an operational perspective have studied the impact of measurable religious phenomena, such as church attendance, Bible reading or denominational preference, on the operational diagnosis of interest. Religious beliefs and practices have been added to other measurable risk or protective factors, such as stressful life events, social support, economic status and hereditary predisposition, in the effort to explain the occurrence of psychiatric disorders. Statistical procedures are employed to quantify the degree to which a psychiatric disorder is caused or prevented by a religious experience or behavior. Religion is thus reduced to a measurable attribute, operationalized through a series of prescribed questions such as

☐ Do you believe in God? (answered "yes" or "no")

☐ Do you attend church services regularly?

☐ Are you a born-again Christian?

Psychiatrists, both Christian and non-Christian, have eagerly accepted this form of investigation, as it parallels other scientific inquiries into the risks for and protectives against psychiatric illness.[46]

Discovering the meaning of questions such as "Do you believe in God?" in survey research is not possible. The dialogue between psychiatry and Christianity thus tends to be reduced to a discussion of statistical association. The statistical association of recovery from depression and the use of an antidepressant medication may convince most psychiatrists and Christians that antidepressants should be prescribed for severe depressions. It is doubtful, though, that an association between the absence of Christian beliefs and the presence of mental illness will convince either psychiatrists or Christians to change their beliefs or practices related to treating emotional suffering. Statistical associations are appealing because they appear to bring understanding and simplicity to an imponderable and complex subject. This simplicity and common sense have influenced psychiatry in yet another way, through cognitive therapies.

The Emergence of Commonsense Psychiatry

Freudian psychoanalysis was the predominant but not the sole force in American psychiatry during the early years of the twentieth century. A key figure in American psychiatry, Adolf Meyer, proposed a commonsense approach to psychiatry. Meyer, from 1910 to 1941 a professor of psychiatry at Johns Hopkins School of Medicine, revolted against the neuropsychiatric view that mental disturbance results from brain pathology alone.[47] Believing that a patient's social environment and disorganized state of thinking are major contributors to the problem, he adopted what he called a psychobiological approach to mental illness. As he distanced himself from the neuropsychiatrists of the nineteenth century, Meyer also kept his distance from psychoanalysts. Specifically, he rejected the idea that psychotherapy should focus on the unconscious. "Your point of reference should always be life itself and not the imagined cesspool of the unconscious."[48] For Meyer, there was no need to distinguish between the unconscious and the conscious. The patient and the psychiatrist each bring a view of the patient's illness to treatment. The goal of treatment should therefore be to approximate these views in a mutually acceptable context, a commonsense approach.

Other psychiatrists were also concerned that psychiatry had wandered too far from common sense. Psychoanalysis was viewed as not being reality-oriented, and the adaptive capacity of the conscious mind was thought to be undermined by psychoanalysis. The dogma of classical psychoanalysis regarded conscious thoughts as only reflections of unconscious conflicts (disguised reflections); therefore the patient's explanations of his or her problem constituted only a defense against any exploration of the real causes of the problem. Psychoanalysis pushed against the grain of the empirical scientific method that guided other medical specialties, and some psychiatrists were becoming concerned that psychiatry had wandered too far from reality.

Aaron Beck picked up this commonsense theme during the middle of the twentieth century and developed perhaps the most popular form of psychotherapy today, cognitive therapy. Beck believed the major schools of psychotherapy had ignored the importance of patients' attempts to solve their problems on their own terms, using their innate rationality.[49] Psychoanalysis attempted to cure neurosis by uncovering hidden or oppressed ideas and translating them into their symbolic meaning. Behavior therapy focused on rewards and punishments for correcting abnormal behaviors and ignored the thoughts of the patient. Neuropsychiatry and psychopharmacology focused on correcting chemical imbalances and ignored psychological causes and cures of emotional suffering. Beck, in contrast, proposed that the core problem in psychiatric disorders, especially depression, is that the psychiatric patient lacks essential information. Depression results largely from irrational thinking based on inadequate information. The psychiatrically disturbed patient therefore experiences thoughts and feelings arising from faulty assumptions.[50] Once adequate information is supplied, common sense can be incorporated to overcome the perceived problem, and the depression will lift.

Cognitive therapy deals with the here and now and does not delve into an individual's past. It does not ask *why* but examines *how* persons think and how these thoughts interfere with emotional well-being. Cognitive therapy is practical, short-term and educational in its approach. Mutual give-and-take occurs between the patient and the therapist as they work to solve the problem. The therapist may assign the patient homework, such as correcting a faulty habit of thinking that diverges from common sense. Negative, irrational beliefs about self, abilities and illness, so-called automatic thoughts, can be overcome once they are identified.

Cognitive therapy is intuitively attractive to me and to many of my colleagues. By its very nature, it requires cooperation between therapist and patient. Control does not rest with the therapist, so control struggles do not become an issue during therapy as much as they might with, for example, behavioral therapies. Since the patient and the cognitive therapist think through the problem together, the patient does not fear thought and behavioral control. Given the concerns about thought control during the 1960s, Beck's therapy could not have emerged at a better time.

In the 1962 novel *A Clockwork Orange* Anthony Burgess describes a young thug, Alex, who is captured by the police and submitted to behavioral therapy in order to control his violent impulses. The therapists come to control him so thoroughly that he submits to every command of his captors, thus totally destroying his independent thoughts and will. Though Alex regains his freedom at the end of the novel, the potential dangers of behavior therapy controlling the will and freedom of persons portrayed in the novel shocked readers worldwide.[51] Cognitive therapy does not conjure up the fears of a behaviorally controlled society elicited by the proposals of the apostle of behavior therapy, B. F. Skinner. In a fictional portrayal of a modern utopia, *Walden II* (1948), Skinner pictured a society in which human problems were solved by scientific control of people's behavior and in which contemporary values of individuality were therefore made obsolete.[52]

It is not surprising that a broad range of mental health professionals and the public have been attracted to cognitive therapy. But does cognitive therapy work? Unlike psychoanalysis, cognitive therapy can be tested in empirical clinical trials, so this question, critical in a cost-conscious society, can potentially be answered.

Psychoanalysis has always been shrouded in mystery because, by its very nature, submitting it to objective evaluation by persons other than the patient and the therapist is almost impossible. The time required for psychoanalysis often extends into years. In addition, there is rarely a comparison therapy against which to determine relative efficacy.

Cognitive therapy, in contrast, can be tested for effectiveness in a manner similar to tests of a medication. The methods are straightforward and can be learned by a therapist in only two or three months of training. Handbooks and training sessions have been developed to ensure that cognitive therapists use virtually identical techniques. Because cognitive therapy usually lasts twelve to twenty-four weeks, patients can be assigned randomly to cognitive therapy or a comparison group. Then the relative improvement of patients undergoing cognitive therapy compared to persons receiving no therapy can be determined. A number of such clinical trials of cognitive therapy have demonstrated it to be more effective than no therapy, and in some cases as effective as medications.

Cognitive therapy is effective and straightforward, yet the above description might suggest the theory underlying cognitive therapy is superficial compared to theories of the traditional psychotherapies. Far from it! Beck, trained in psychoanalysis, is one of the most creative and thoughtful persons in modern psychiatry. When he began to develop cognitive therapy, he was reacting in large part to the psychiatric community's unwillingness to take the time to test whether psychoanalysis and other "depth psychologies" were effective. Furthermore, professional cognitive therapists are neither uncaring or unskilled. In fact, cognitive therapists are empathic, sensitive persons who weave their own intuitive and interpersonal skills into the framework of cognitive theory and therapy.

Cognitive therapy is not the only here-and-now, commonsense therapy. Interpersonal psychotherapy (IPT) is another popular therapy for depression.[53] This time-limited treatment focuses on interpersonal behavior rather than cognition or intrapsychic phenomena. The therapist identifies one of four interpersonal problems from which depressed persons usually suffer:

grief, disputes with close friends or relatives, role transitions and interpersonal problems that lead to isolation, and loneliness. Once a primary problem is identified, the therapist concentrates on helping the patient understand the problem and suggesting ways to overcome it. Emphasis is placed on the patient's ability to control, and thereby improve, interpersonal relations through rational discussions of relations with the therapist. The theory underlying IPT is similar to that behind cognitive therapy. Cognitive therapy thus serves as the prototype for a new wave of therapies which have arisen in reaction to psychoanalysis and have been readily appropriated by the Christian community, as described in chapter four.

The pragmatic appeal of commonsense therapy does not address one question of relevance to the interface between psychiatry and Christianity: How does psychotherapy heal? This question, unlike empirical studies, necessarily addresses the theories and values underlying a particular therapy. I believe therapists firmly embedded in a faith tradition need to carefully examine the underlying values and the methods of the form of therapy they use.

Though I find it most comfortable to practice cognitive therapy, I am frequently uncomfortable with the context in which I practice it. My discomfort is not easy to explain and requires a paradigm for examining the therapy quite different from empirical science. I have selected a paradigm for an examination of cognitive therapy which places the therapy in context. My goal is not that readers critique the paradigm (there are many others that could be applied), and I would like not to be held to the conclusions I draw (I may have changed my views by the time you read this book!). Rather, I ask you to follow the process of exploring a popular therapy within the context of culture and cultural/religious values.

Examining Cognitive Therapy

Arthur Kleinman has reviewed crosscultural and ethnographic data and developed a paradigm of healing within the context of culture.[54] How does cognitive therapy fit this paradigm? How do modern Western society's beliefs and symbols mold cognitive therapy? Kleinman suggests that four structural processes are essential for accomplishing symbolic healing. The first process or stage posits the presence of a symbolic bridge between personal experience, social relations and cultural meanings. Individuals orient themselves to a group's symbols. Among traditional Christians, for example, emotional suffering or misfortune might be oriented to the crucified Christ.[55] Healing in the traditional Christian community would therefore be oriented to the power of the resurrected Christ to relieve or identify with one's suffering.

Cognitive therapy does not appear to orient itself to a particular set of symbols—or does it? The commonsense approach to psychotherapy fits well into the religious climate today in Western society. First, though no modern Western country is more openly religious than the United States, Harold Bloom, in his book *The American Religion*, suggests that Americans do not typically perceive religion as coming close to them as individuals.[56] Concern with guilt, death, pain and suffering has largely disappeared from religious conversations in American society, especially among evangelical Christians. Based on my experience as a therapist who has treated many professing Christians, I believe Bloom is correct. The self is not so much oriented to the crucified Christ as Christ has been oriented to the self. In other words, Christ can be appropriated for healing: "Christ helps those who help themselves." Therefore the religious in our society, especially evangelical Christians, believe it to be a sign of their faith to call on their own resources for healing. The symbolic bridge between individual suffering and the Christian faith is, for many, embedded in the American belief in individualism, self-sufficiency, pragmatism and realism.[57]

Stage two of Kleinman's thesis begins with the symbolic connection of personal experience with societal symbols activated for the person.[58] The therapist persuades the patient that the problem from which she or he suffers can be redefined in terms of the authorizing system of meaning. In the case of cognitive therapy, the problem is defined in terms of illogical assumptions based on lack of information. The accumulation of accurate information and use of logic to assess this information will naturally lead to healing. Information has become the currency for power and success in our society. Cognitive therapy leaves little room for the person whose emotions are so severely disturbed, as with severe depression or schizophrenia, that information and logic cannot overcome the pain of the emotions. Cognitive therapy leaves little room for the patient to say, "I have every reason to feel depressed or fearful." Though Beck would not impose positive thinking on the tragic, therapists trained in cognitive therapy often are frustrated in the face of tragedy.

The modern evangelical Christian also appeals to knowledge of Scripture and inherent logic in order to overcome virtually every problem of living. In contrast, the Judeo-Christian heritage provided a powerful authorizing system for understanding and accepting human suffering in the person of Jesus, who experienced persecution, ridicule, misunderstanding and ultimately crucifixion. Logic was deemphasized, as exemplified in the Bible's account of the suffering of Job. When Job appealed to God for an explanation as to why he was afflicted with such emotional and physical pain, God provided no logical explanation but asked, "Where were you when I laid the earth's foundation? Tell me, if you understand. . . . I will question you, and you will answer me" (Job 38:4; 40:7). As described in chapter two, theodicy, the attempt to explain (or explain away) evil and human suffering, is a relatively new phenomenon in the history of the Christian church.

During Kleinman's third stage, the healer guides change in the patient's emotional reactions through mediating symbols applied to the patient from the general system of meaning within the culture. For example, in psychoanalysis the anxiety an individual patient experiences is interpreted as a reexperiencing of the culturally universal anxiety of the Oedipus complex. When the individual recognizes the universal anxiety, his or her personal anxiety is relieved. In cognitive therapy the therapist encourages the patient to practice logical "rethinking." For example, the therapist may ask, "What do you want to do about your depression: make it better or make it worse?"

The patient answers, "Make it better."

The therapist then may ask, "How does criticizing yourself or being depressed lighten your depression?"

The patient responds, "It won't."

Then the therapist suggests that rather than criticizing oneself, perhaps the patient should look for some new approach to overcome the depression. Depression, according to the cognitive therapist, is not an existential experience to be shared but a puzzle to be solved, an unknown to be known.

Problem-solving as a mediating symbol is appealing to both psychiatrists and modern Christian counselors and creates little conflict between psychiatry and Christianity. It provides a common language that does not challenge the Christian faith, since faith rarely becomes a topic of discussion in cognitive therapy. At the same time it appeals to what both the psychiatrist and the Christian counselor believe actually matters in day-to-day experience—collecting data and making logical decisions based on those data. Yet experiential rather than logical understanding has been the historical mediation between sufferings Christian and their God.

Kleinman's last stage consists of the healer's confirming the transformation of a specific symbolic meaning in the interruption of personal events.[59] In other words, healing occurs in part as the experience of emotional suffering is interpreted as meaningful. Cognitive therapy paradoxically robs suffering of its meaning. The goal of cognitive psychotherapy is expressed in the title of two popular books on modern psychotherapy—*I'm OK, You're OK*[60] and *Feeling Good*. Of course, virtually all persons who suffer painful emotions wish to believe they are OK and to feel good. Yet many never achieve this goal and ask, "Why me? Why must I continue to suffer?" Others who do recover ask, "Why did this happen to me?" Cognitive therapy renders these questions irrelevant to its purpose if the answer cannot be readily identified. Both pastoral care and evangelical Christian counseling have typically framed these questions as does the cognitive therapist, by asking, "What is happening to this person psychologically which explains the overt spiritual or existential struggle?" Rarely is the spiritual or existential struggle itself seen to be central to the problem. At this very point popular writers such as Scott Peck and Thomas Moore have sought to fill the vacuum, but their efforts spring from neither mainline modern psychiatry nor modern pastoral care or Christian counseling. (See below and chapter six.)

Psychiatry Finds Its Identity But Loses Its Soul

During the past twenty-five years, psychiatry has taken great strides in establishing its identity. Though not the most popular of medical specialties, psychiatry has emerged as a legitimate specialty with a solid scientific base. By focusing on the more seriously ill, such as the schizophrenic, the manic-depressive, the severe depressive and the obsessive-compulsive, psychiatry has undertaken the study and treatment of problems that few deny deserve the attention of a physician. Psychiatrists are much less likely to treat the worried well today than during midcentury. The techniques used by psychiatrists—the diagnostic interview, the laboratory and new pharmacotherapies—parallel traditional medical therapies. Even current psychotherapies, such as cognitive therapy, have their parallel in physical medicine. For example, current treatment of the diabetic includes a commonsense educational program regarding lifestyle as well as the prescription of insulin. Yet psychiatry is now attracting fewer graduating medical students than in years past. Some suggest psychiatry has lost its vitality.

I want to suggest that the problem is not that psychiatry is without mind, but rather that it is without soul. The very concept of soul is difficult for the psychiatrist to grasp, because it defies definition. Too often the discussion of soul leads to debate such as whether the dualism of Plato, separating the soul from the body and empowering it with transcendent properties, is an appropriate construct for exploring the mental life of persons. Even so, the concept of soul strikes most of us intuitively as representing wholeness, depth and meaning beyond chemical messengers, empirical science and common sense. Thomas Moore, in his popular book *Care of the Soul,* says:

> The great malady of the twentieth century, implicated in all of our troubles and affecting us individually and socially, is "loss of soul." . . . It is impossible to define precisely what the soul is . . . [yet] we say certain music has soul or a remarkable person is soulful. . . . Soul is revealed in attachment, love and community, as well as in retreat.[61]

Jeffrey Boyd, a psychiatrist and Episcopal minister, insists that psychiatrists treat the soul whether they acknowledge soul in therapy or not: "If psychiatrists and psychologists treat the whole person or the whole personality, then the focus of their treatment is on the soul. . . . If therapists treat mental illness, such as depression or schizophrenia, they would be understood in biblical times to be treating evil spirits that invade the soul from outside."[62]

I believe modern psychiatry has lost its own soul as it has drifted from concerns about wholeness, meaning and the transcendent. Psychiatrists are much less inclined to converse among themselves or with their patients about soul than earlier in the twentieth century. We may treat the soul, yet we often behave as if we are no longer soul mates with our patients.

I began this chapter by describing my frustration with the barriers which have arisen between me and my patients. I have necessarily changed my practice style as psychiatry has changed over the past twenty-five years. I have become a better doctor in many ways. In the past I spent countless hours working with patients whom I knew I could not help but to whom I felt obligated to continue to "relate" in a nonconfrontational style—a remnant of my training in psychodynamic psychiatry. It cost me time and cost them both time and money, for no apparent purpose. I rarely find myself locked in such relationships today. The changes described above have prevented me from entering into relationships that are not therapeutic and encouraged me to use medications, often with dramatic results, when listening and talking are to no avail.

Yet I believe my patients and I have lost as much as we have gained. I don't know them, they don't know me, and psychiatry is frankly just not as rewarding. I have withdrawn my soul in large part from my practice.

4

Christianity Loses Its Mind

My *maternal grandfather and* grandmother were about as conservative as any American Christians in the early twentieth century. He was an elder and song leader in a noninstrumental, fundamentalist Church of Christ near Nashville, Tennessee, and she was an English teacher at a local high school. My grandfather worked as a mail carrier and never completed high school. They died before I could have memories of either of them. Yet I feel I know them well, for I inherited many of their books. Both were avid readers and made numerous marginal notes in the books that have come into my possession.

These semirural, southern fundamental Christians viewed acceptance of the doctrine and practices of their faith tradition as an intellectual challenge, and they could provide a logical, even philosophical, argument for virtually everything they believed and practiced. If they had been alive when I entered psychiatry, I have no doubt we would have engaged in some long and heated discussions about the underlying values and philosophy of this new "mind therapy." From what I have heard, they both welcomed a friendly debate. I suspect they would have challenged the writings of Freud, but they would have been familiar with them. They were distressed by the emergence of liberal theology in the early twentieth century, but they understood liberal theology. My grandparents were not only faithful but thoughtful Christians. I suspect they would be most disappointed in the mindlessness of many of our Christian conversations today, especially with the rise of the Christian counseling industry.

It seems to me that Christianity has lost its mind. If my grandparents are at all representative, then even among the most conservative Christians early in the twentieth century, some thoughtful persons were not reticent to question their own beliefs and practices even as they challenged others. I rarely find people like my grandparents in my faith tradition today. So I often return to reading the marginal notes in the books I inherited.

The Fundamentalist Reaction to Liberal Theology

As the changes in psychiatry over the past twenty-five years have roots in nineteenth-century neuropsychiatry, recent changes that have occurred in Christian counseling have roots in the early twentieth century. These roots lie, to a significant extent, in the evangelical reaction to liberal theology and the positive thinking movement. The 1960s were the turning point for Christian counseling in the United States.

To understand the current trends in Christian counseling and pastoral care, one must appreciate the impact of the 1960s on Bible-believing and church-attending Christians. Some labeled the 1960s as the decade of the "death of God" or of the "Great Moral Revolution."[1] Though doubts had arisen prior to the 1960s regarding the United States's role as moral leader of the world, the moral tradition of the country had been widely perceived as intact. Few could deny, however, that the changes that occurred during the 1960s severely weakened that tradition. The culture's dominant themes shifted. One of these shifts involved rapid secularization, as exhibited in actions of the Supreme Court. In 1963 religious ceremonies were declared unconstitutional in schools, thus undermining the perceived connection of evangelical Christians' faith and public education. Yet the events of the 1960s had roots that reached back through several decades.

Early in the twentieth century, some Christians were busy with Bible conferences and revivals, whereas others had turned their attention to reversing social ills such as industrialization and corporate profits.[2] By 1920 many Christians felt a need to return to the fundamentals of the faith while almost simultaneously the "social gospel," as a movement, gained strength. Much of the tension between conservative fundamentalists (such as my grandparents) and liberal proponents of the social gospel centered on questions of whether religion and science (both biological and social science) could coexist. Fundamentalists tended to be uneducated but were thoroughly grounded in the logical thought style of the Enlightenment. Liberal theology, however, dominated the divinity schools of the best-known educational institutions and mainline Protestant Christianity. Though liberal theologians were well aware of and discussed Freud and psychoanalysis, fundamentalists concentrated their arguments on defending the church from the perceived threat of evolutionary biology, which they associated with communism and other social ills. Freud was of only peripheral concern to them.

Fundamentalist and anti-intellectual themes flourished in Protestant Christianity briefly after World War I. The liberal theology that challenged the authenticity of the Scriptures, coupled with a progressive and pragmatic social gospel, filled many Christians with anxiety and even a sense of betrayal. Years before Jerry Falwell, spokespersons such as William Jennings Bryan expressed their concerns about dominant themes in Protestant Christianity. The most visible example of this reaction to the mainline church was the effort to prevent public schools and universities from teaching evolution for its perceived incompatibility with a traditional interpretation of the Bible.[3]

This effort reached its climax in 1925 during the trial of John Scopes in Dayton, Tennessee. Bryan argued for the prosecution, and Clarence Darrow defended Scopes, who was tried for teaching evolution in the local school. Though the trial itself was more a show of the oratorical skills of Bryan and Darrow (and a field day for newspaper reporters), the event awakened a sleeping giant in Protestant Christianity, especially in the South.

The Scopes trial itself turned into a disaster for the fundamentalists, as the battle against evolution became only sporadic and remained on the fringes of even the most conservative churches until mid-twentieth century. Early in the century, fundamentalist attacks on Darwin embarrassed and weakened the movement, and the carnival atmosphere at the Scopes trial contributed significantly to that embarrassment. Creationism was equated with the ignorant dirt farmer of the culturally backward South. A revitalization of "creation science" would not occur until the 1960s.[4]

Creation science is based on a literal interpretation of the book of Genesis and claims that the world's history can be measured in thousands rather than billions of years. Though not accepted by the scientific community at large, a group of evangelicals, both theologians and scientists, developed a theory that they believe explains most geological phenomena in concert with the universal flood described in the book of Genesis. The best known of their published works is *The Genesis Flood* (1961), written by John C. Whitcomb Jr. and Henry Morris and published by Baker Book House, a conservative Christian publishing company. Whitcomb was a minister and Morris a hydraulics engineer, trained at Rice University, who later served as chair of an engineering department at Virginia Tech University.

The history of scientific creationism parallels in some respects the history of the evangelical Christian counseling movement, for both gained their impetus from a reaction to secular scholarship, sought to address the evangelical church member more than the scientific community, and developed parallel to their secular counterparts rather than in meaningful dialogue with them. Differences emerged, however. Scientific creationists never gained widespread acceptance among evangelicals and continually sought to engage a debate with secular biologists and geologists to gain credibility. The Christian counseling movement attracted far more adherents, and its leaders have not been nearly as interested in engaging psychiatry or secular psychology in dialogue or debate.

Mainline Protestant churches have also reacted to liberal theological scholarship. Their reaction derived from a struggle for control of the church. Liberal theologians were clearly in control of mainline Protestant churches during the first part of the century. For the most part, churches in the South were not threatened. The Southern Baptist Convention was always a home for the most conservative elements of Christianity. Many battles ensued among Southern Baptists, yet its conservatives and moderates were more likely to engage a battle with one another than with liberals. The tension in the Northern Baptist Convention, in contrast, was profound.[5] Despite the fact that the Baptist church grew predominantly by revivalism among the uneducated, many of the best educated liberal theologians were Baptist, including Walter Rauschenbusch and Harry Emerson Fosdick. One outcome of this struggle was that Baptist conservatives were able to persuade their fellows against continuing membership in the interchurch world movement in 1920. Conservatives withdrew unto themselves.

During the 1930s conservative, revivalistic Christian groups grew rapidly throughout the United States.[6] Many Bible institutes were established to compete directly with seminaries associated with universities, and the mass media were used effectively to reach the public. For example, Charles E. Fuller broadcast the *Old-Fashioned Revival Hour* most successfully from Los Angeles. The heart of the conflict was liberal theologians' perceived challenge to biblical inerrancy. An anti-intellectual seed began to flower among conservatives during those early decades of the twentieth century in parallel with the reaction to liberal theology. My grandparents would not have appreciated the full flowering of this trend. Many intellectuals left Protestant Christianity. H. L. Mencken railed:

> Any literate plowhead, if the Holy Spirit inflames him, is thought to be fit to preach. Is he commonly sent . . . to college? But what a college! You will find one in every mountain and valley of the land. . . . One man in such a college teaches oratory, ancient history, arithmetic and Old Testament exegesis.[7]

The fundamentalists appeared to react against everything modern, not just biblical criticism, the theory of evolution and the social gospel. They were noticeably averse to inquiring into the history of Christianity. Instead they emphasized the restoration of the New Testament church in the twentieth century, virtually ignoring two thousand years of church history.

The Ascendance of Evangelicalism
Even as liberal theologians and pastors were engaging psychiatrists and psychologists in conversations centering on pastoral care, they were losing

the attention of members of their churches to an emerging conservative Christian group, the evangelicals. The most significant strength of the evangelicals was their ability to attract the attention of Protestants who felt alienated from both church and state. Fundamentalists had proved ineffectual in changing the content of science taught in schools and lost out in most political battles over such issues. Even universities that had been historically controlled by more fundamental religious groups became increasingly secular from the 1920s to the 1960s. For example, traditional Baptist schools such as Baylor University and Wake Forest University emerged as seats of liberalism. Therefore, evangelical leaders worked to ensure that liberal Protestant Christianity and the theologians identified with it would not maintain control over the religious beliefs and activities of evangelical Christians in the United States.

Mainline Protestant churches consequently lost much of their intellectual and literary leadership in society as a whole and among their own members, for the energy and growth within the Christian community during the last few decades has been among evangelicals.[8] The Christian counseling industry of the later twentieth century has taken full advantage of the energy of the new evangelicals and the reaction against liberal Protestant theology.

As fundamentalism faded as an influence and evangelicals gained strength, the anti-intellectual thrust was less visible, though it did not disappear. Many evangelical leaders studied at excellent institutions of higher learning and subsequently developed a more sophisticated theology. The Bible colleges described by Mencken evolved, in many cases, into accredited liberal arts colleges during the middle decades of the twentieth century. Yet the instructors in these colleges, even today, have not typically joined with colleagues from their disciplines in secular universities, especially in disciplines where conflict emerged between evangelical beliefs and the current themes dominating secular scholarship. Mark Noll, a professor of Christian thought at Wheaton College, has bemoaned the current lack of rigorous thought among evangelicals in his book *The Scandal of the Evangelical Mind.*[9]

Noll suggests that the lack of scholarship among evangelicals has been especially noticeable in the sciences. This has been no more true than in the field of counseling and psychology. Most professors in evangelical colleges who teach psychology and counseling have been trained in secular institutions, yet they focus primarily on teaching and practice rather than research. They are more apt to write books for popular consumption than to contribute to the scientific literature or maintain an ongoing relationship with their secular colleagues at scientific meetings. Unlike their secular colleagues, they have not made it a priority to explore the frontiers of psychiatry, psychology and the neurosciences. Rather, they have been content to pick up new findings in their disciplines secondhand. This educational orientation took root during the 1940s and 1950s and has changed little to this day. Within my own faith community, the faculties of our Christian colleges remain relatively isolated from secular scholarship.

For me as an evangelical Christian, this educational approach had some appeal. During my training as a psychiatrist I seriously considered moving to a community that housed one of these Christian colleges. I imagined a comfortable and productive life, splitting my responsibilities across practicing psychiatry primarily among evangelical Christians, supervising ministers as they counseled church members and teaching undergraduate courses in psychology and religion. (Many of my psychiatric colleagues from evangelical Christian backgrounds did what I imagined I would do.) This life would have left little room for ongoing relationships with secular psychiatrists and certainly no room for psychiatric investigation.

During the 1950s evangelicals grew dramatically in number. At least three factors contributed to this growth. First, the tremendous success of the Billy Graham evangelistic crusades during the 1950s assured that the evangelical message became known throughout the world. Second, evangelical groups penetrated secular universities during the sixties. Evangelical unions, such as InterVarsity Christian Fellowship, provided students a means to explore the implications of their faith apart from the traditional courses in religion offered by universities. Third, many bright and energetic young persons, perhaps attracted by Graham's success, sought ministry positions in evangelical congregations as a viable and attractive profession.[10] Therefore, when the challenges to traditional beliefs by Bishop J. A. T. Robinson, Harvey Cox and Thomas Altizer became public, an army of evangelicals was ready to strike back at these challenges and to mobilize millions of confused and alienated Protestants.

Many Americans sought to reestablish their religious identity during the turbulent 1960s. These persons felt the need to return to their roots and find secure answers to the tough questions the sixties posed. Evangelical Christianity provided many of these answers through a return to the faith in opposition to modernism. This return assumed a militant and revolutionary character. Evangelical Christians, like militant revolutionists, deemphasized centuries of intervening history as they attempted to reestablish the vision of first-century Christianity by restoring old beliefs and values. This countermovement to mainline Protestantism is best exemplified in the Jesus Movement among young people of the 1960s and early 1970s. They disdained church (and therefore historical) authority, took Jesus as a personal example and worked for peace and social justice. They stressed love and tried to rescue persons who had fallen victim to the excesses of the 1960s, especially the drug culture.

By the 1960s fundamentalist Christianity, as a movement, had largely been replaced by evangelical Christianity. The evangelicalism that emerged never viewed itself as departing from the "fundamentals" of the faith. Yet it did seek to change its image from a reactionary, confrontational movement to one that provided answers to real-life problems. Carl F. H. Henry wrote in 1947 that the thrust of new evangelicalism "is not . . . troubled about the great biblical truths but rather . . . distressed by the frequent failure to apply them effectively to critical problems confronting the modern mind."[11] The evangelical movement, however, established its epistemological base on a belief in Scripture's clarity as well as its authority.

Forty million Americans were thought to be evangelicals during the 1960s. (Today evangelicals are estimated to number over seventy million in the United States.) In 1969 Billy Graham wrote, "I think evangelical Christianity is now 'where the action is.'"[12] Not only was Graham preaching to hundreds of thousands every year, membership in evangelical churches had increased from 400 to 700 percent during the two decades following World War II, in contrast to 75 to 90 percent for the older Protestant denominations.[13] The initial evangelical emphases were on conservative doctrine and foreign missions, yet evangelicals were also primed to reach out to the many Americans who were "unchurched" or felt alienated from mainline Protestant churches. Providing clear biblical answers to problems of daily living was a potent method for evangelism, and therefore an industry of Christian counseling arose from evangelical Christianity to parallel the pastoral counseling movement of the mainline Protestant churches. Yet the epistemological roots of evangelical Christian counseling were decidedly different from those of pastoral counseling, just as the epistemological roots of evangelical Christianity were different from those of liberal Protestant Christianity.

Central among the basic tenets of evangelicalism that have shaped Christian counseling is the emphasis on a spiritually transformed life. The sole authority in religion is the Bible, and the sole means of salvation is a life-transforming experience facilitated by the Holy Spirit through faith in Jesus Christ. Evangelical Christian counseling therefore developed from a context that deemphasized theology and traditional psychotherapy explicitly. Christian counseling was by nature practical and emphasized change within a short period of time toward the transformed life. The Bible's authority implied its usefulness as a practical guidebook for living. Scriptures were sprinkled frequently through counseling books and counseling sessions. The less a Christian counselor referred to the work of a secular psychologist or psychiatrist the better.

In parallel, I have found that individual evangelical Christians express little interest in exploring their personal histories in the context of the religious communities in which they reside. When I first encounter Christians in therapy, they rarely wish to discuss their spiritual journey in the faith. Jason, for example, had no more interest in understanding the context of the emotional pain he experienced than he would have wished to understand his life history as a context for a sore toe (see chapter one). Confession and life review have been deemphasized. Modern evangelical Christians want to feel good about the here and now, and the evangelical Christian counseling industry has supported this view.

Literary critic Harold Bloom, in his book *The American Religion,* defines the prototypical American form of religious expression as evangelical

Christianity, a religion fiercely searching for "the spirit." Yet that spirit is not necessarily the spirit of the transcendent God.[14] The actual (though hidden) agenda of American religion is inner freedom, an affirmation of the spirit of self. The American religion does not encourage community or confession, because the individualism of American society drives its religion toward inner solitude. Evangelicals focus on the resurrected rather than the crucified Jesus and therefore envision a revitalized rather than suffering self. Just as the Gnostics of the first two centuries of the Christian era sought to know their inner spirit and unite that spirit with the divine light, salvation for the evangelical does not come through community or congregational confession but through a personal and private relationship with Jesus.

Most of the patients I treat from evangelical faith traditions tend to float from one congregation to another. If problems arise with fellow church members (and they are very likely to arise if a person is experiencing emotional pain), the easiest solution is to move to another congregation, perhaps even commit oneself to a different (though not dramatically different) set of beliefs. Recall that Jason made a significant move from one faith community to another with little thought given to the loss of support and community relations (see chapter one). Within the evangelical community, one may float across a sea of slight variations in doctrine and scores of congregations of Christians. This phenomenon is incomprehensible to my Jewish friends when I describe it to them. Faith for the Jew means attachment to the community, to Israel, through a long and tortured history. Faith cannot be separated from community or history. Yet for the troubled evangelical, the perception of isolation from any religious tradition or community is all too common an experience.

During the 1960s evangelical Christians had little interest in psychiatry or the psychology of religion. These Christians instead were mounting parallel and paradoxical campaigns for individual self-sufficiency and conservative Christianity as a remedy for damaged emotions, as described by Robert Bellah and colleagues in *Habits of the Heart:*

> Radically individualistic religion, particularly when it takes the form of a belief in cosmic self-hood, may seem to be in a different world from conservative or fundamentalist religion. Yet these are two poles that

organize much of American religious life. To the first, God is simply the self magnified; and to the second, God confronts man from outside the universe. One seeks a self that is finally identical with the world; the other seeks an external God who will provide order in the world. Both value personal experience as a basis of their belief.[15]

The Bible has become the symbol of the absolute and inviolate transcendent God confronting humanity from outside the universe. And interestingly, evangelicals' insistence on biblical inerrancy does not necessarily mean they practice sustained reading of Scripture.[16] They are more likely to use the Bible as a weapon or justification than as a stimulus to explore their own lives. The Bible has been converted into an icon, and from this icon the industry of Christian counseling has in part emerged. As suggested below, evangelical Christian counseling does not so much derive from biblical theology as use biblical inerrancy to validate its predominantly cognitive, rational, self-sufficient, positivistic message. By sprinkling passages of Scripture throughout pop psychology books, Christian writers assert their credibility within the evangelical community regardless of their message.

In retrospect, I believe I remained in secular academic psychiatry for two reasons. First, my perception of the central role of the Christian's sacred journey through her or his emotional suffering was often not shared by the Christian patients I treated. They had little desire to explore their faith through time. Rather they wanted me to make their faith work, to make it chase away the pain. Perhaps by special prayer, perhaps by laying on of healing hands, perhaps by a prescription of behavior that would guarantee financial success or a happy marriage, I, the Christian psychiatrist, was expected to mediate a quick healing. Though I would never limit God, I knew my limits. I am *not* a charismatic healer.

Second, that comfortable faith community was more apparent than real. I learned that churches, Christian colleges and congregations of evangelical Christians were often as conflicted as the secular university where I was training. I recognized that my family and I must work to make our local faith community as strong as possible. To contribute to strengthening that community, I had to join it not as a specialist but as an equal partner. Rather than be "the church psychiatrist," I felt more comfortable and productive as

a church member who happened to be a psychiatrist, not unlike my friend
and brother who happens to be a transportation engineer.

Attempts to Integrate Psychiatry into Christianity

Prior to and concurrent with the rise of the Christian counseling industry,
there were attempts to reconcile psychiatry and Christianity from within the
evangelical Christian community. These attempts were launched by persons
who were firmly grounded in their faith and spoke primarily to the Christian
community. In contrast to the mental health professionals and theologians
described in chapter two, these persons truly worked at the interface of
psychiatry and Christianity. One of the best known attempts was initiated
by Paul Tournier, a Swiss physician.[17] Though not trained in psychiatry,
Tournier elected to practice psychiatry. He did not contribute extensively to
the psychiatric literature, was not university-based and was virtually unknown to secular psychiatrists. He was a clinician with a strong Christian
faith who felt impelled to write to Christians about the experiences of his
patients as they groped to find their God. Psychotherapeutic healing for
Tournier necessarily involved an exploration of the relationship between the
patient and God. His warm and accepting style appealed to both liberal and
conservative Christians.

Based firmly in traditional psychotherapy at mid-twentieth century,
Tournier nevertheless demonstrated unique insights that reflected his spiri-
tual approach to therapy. For example, in his book *The Meaning of Persons*
Tournier took pains to integrate body and soul for the reader:

> Spiritual life involves the whole person, and not only the psychological
> processes studied by psychologists. . . . If the frontier between psychol-
> ogy and the life of the spirit is hard to define, nevertheless in crossing it
> we enter a completely different domain: that of judgments, of values, of
> faith, of decisions involving self-commitment.[18]

Tournier goes on to suggest that sickness of soul, such as that caused by
depression, distorts and hinders growth of relationships with God and
others.

Within his psychiatric practice, Tournier observed God relating with
people to free their souls of disease and join with them to heal the whole

person. "With a patient we work for weeks—even months—on end, in utter darkness, and suddenly light shines—the living God has been breaking in upon that person."[19]

What set Tournier apart from many evangelical Christians who practice psychiatry is that he did not perceive a need to Christianize psychiatry nor to psychologize Christianity. The ease with which he moved from his consultation room to the Bible and back again, the gentle and supportive approach to his patients and the firm conviction of the healing power of biblical faith are worthy examples of the potential for conversation between psychiatry and evangelical Christianity.

Tournier did not, however, explore the difficult theological and moral issues that tend to divide psychiatry and Christianity. For him there was little to debate. He virtually ignored neuropsychiatry, despite his medical training. When he did discuss difficult theological or philosophical problems, he was inclined to take the middle road. For example, when considering the doctor's right to use psychotherapy to change personality, he presented the case for and against such practice but did not suggest a solution to the dilemma. In discussing the use of lobotomy, the severing of connections between the frontal lobe and the remainder of the brain (a procedure now largely considered barbaric), Tournier took a surprisingly accommodating position. "To condemn every interference with the personality would be to condemn the whole of medicine. . . . To draw a hard-and-fast line anywhere between them is to engage in arbitrary casuistry."[20]

Another attempt to integrate psychiatry and Christianity during the 1950s was made by Albert Outler in *Psychotherapy and the Christian Message.*[21] Outler, a respected Protestant theologian, spoke to the growth and evolution of pastoral care rather than evangelical Christian counseling. Nevertheless, a review of his concerns provides an important context for the rise of Christian counseling. He began with the premise that modern psychotherapy is more than just another development of the healing arts: it is a challenge to, as well as an opportunity for, Christian thought. He recognized the common goals of the two fields, especially in regard to the practical aspects of interpersonal relations and unresolved intrapersonal conflicts: "The problem has been prematurely solved in many ways, ranging from outright rejection from one side or the other to amiable agreements to ignore theory as far as possible and to concentrate on the practical matters."[22]

Even during the early 1950s, Outler recognized the trend that would dominate evangelical counseling—practical solutions divorced from theology. Outler was not content with these practical solutions. Though Christianity and modern psychiatry were both "wisdom about life, it was by no means clear that they were the same wisdom. Psychotherapeutic exploration must recognize that one must have a foundation from which to explore. For myself, I have chosen and confirmed the Christian faith as the primary source of whatever wisdom there may be in these pages."[23]

Outler thus not only noted that all psychotherapies were based on a value system but also clearly stated his own values. He recognized the inherent tension between psychiatry and Christianity. According to Outler, given that psychoanalysis reduces Christianity to an obsession that cannot be proven by modern scientific methods, psychiatry naturally is prejudiced against Christianity. That places the Christian in a compromised position. "Even to argue with a psychotherapist who reduces Christian proclamations to perverted, psychological material is to weaken the Christian position . . . to treat the unfaith of the pagan seriously."[24] Nevertheless, Outler accepted the practical, empirical wisdom of psychiatry regarding relationships via certain principles of secular psychotherapy: the respect for persons inherent in the therapeutic relationship; the discovery that behavior is not really meaningless and should never be dismissed simply as unintelligible; the therapeutic process itself, especially the art of listening; a life-course perspective, from infancy to old age; and the possibility that religious thought can be used in a delusional and protective way.

Outler warned the Christian that fear of scientifically based psychiatry is at times justified. The scientist who does succeed in describing and controlling natural processes will frequently overreach the limitations of scientific method and claim that "what is not science is not knowledge." "The Christian faith can assimilate any scientific claim save one: the claim that omnicompetence of science is scientific and verifiable."[25]

Outler also challenged the psychiatrist. "Their charge, that religious faith in God is a projection of infantile wishes upon the cosmos, is not free from its own projective aspects. Theism is man's acknowledgment of radical dependence upon God and his finitely-free responsibility as creature and citizen of God's beloved community."[26] What sets Outler apart from evangelical critics of psychiatry is his nonsectarian, nonaggressive challenge to psychiatry:

> Christianity has neither the right, nor the power, to displace or eliminate the reigning naturalism in psychotherapy by fiat or decree. It has no right—and, I should hope, no desire—to foster a rival psychotherapy which is merely tailored to fit the dogmas and traditions of historic Christianity. . . . It has the right to ask of psychotherapy that its prevailing presuppositions be reviewed at a new level of self-critical inquiry.[27]

Outler recognized that psychiatry and Christianity must divide their labor, but he called on them to synthesize their goals. He believed that a psychiatrist can work as effectively with assumptions and goals derived from the Christian faith as with secular scientific presuppositions. Christians can therefore enter psychiatry and practice it effectively.

At the time Outler published his book, few professing Christians, even fewer evangelical Christians, had entered psychiatry as a profession. During the past twenty-five years, however, many Christians have obtained professional training in psychiatry. This in part can be explained by the move among evangelicals to become better educated, but it also reflects the decreased tension between psychiatry and Christianity. Unfortunately, most Christian professionals have not been inclined to explore the tough theoretical issues with their secular colleagues the way Outler encouraged us to do. Rather, evangelical Christians entering psychiatry either became incorporated into mainstream psychiatry or joined the emerging industry of Christian counseling. This industry was initially fueled by Christian counselors' writing popular books, putting on large seminars, developing a distinctive professional identity and entering the political arena.

The Popularization of Christian Counseling

The roots of evangelical Christian counseling in the commonsense therapies of Adolf Meyer, Aaron Beck and others are clear. Yet these roots also extend back to practical guidebooks earlier in the twentieth century, such as

Norman Vincent Peale's *The Power of Positive Thinking.*[28] The most popular Christian counselors have focused on practical advice in their books and seminars, as opposed to exploring the theological and philosophical relation of Christianity and psychiatry. These counselors rarely leave thorny problems open for discussion, at least on the surface of their work. Their practical and frequently dogmatic prescriptions for healing and success do not apply to the most distressed among us, those with whom psychiatrists must work. I am commonly asked at my church to recommend a "good book" for a person struggling with a severe problem. Rarely can I identify a book that speaks to the needs of persons deeply distressed. Popular Christian books are tailored instead to the healthy and serve more to boost confidence than to confront the realities of serious emotional suffering.

Popular Christian counselors have not directed their attention to the severely mentally ill. The boundary between advice from a pastor and professional Christian counseling is blurred, yet the characteristics of popular Christian counseling are clear. Pastors such as Tim LaHaye do not hesitate to promise their readers advice on "how to win over depression."[29] James Mallory, an evangelical psychiatrist, speaks to the everyday problems of evangelical Christians in *The Kink and I: A Psychiatrist's Guide to Untwisted Living.*[30] These writers have become popular because they address the everyday problems experienced by evangelicals, not the more complex problems of the mentally ill.

Gary Collins has identified nine elements common to popular Christian counseling: relevance, simplicity, practicality, avoidance of the academic, communication skills, personal appeal, biblical orientation, reactionary nature and uniqueness.[31] These elements are manifested in popular writings, seminars and conferences as much as in individual counseling sessions. For example, even when the Christian counseling industry was in its early stages, Bill Gothard's seminar on "basic youth conflicts" attracted over 250,000 persons in 1973.[32] Gothard speaks primarily to Christians who are psychologically healthy and who he believes can benefit spiritually. He emphasizes living the Christian life, keeping the rules and thereby gaining the joy of knowing one is doing right.

Popular counseling was not unique to evangelical Christianity, for during the late 1960s and early 1970s many secular psychiatrists and psychologists wrote popular books. Among them were Eric Berne's *Games People Play,* Fritz Perls's *Gestalt Therapy Verbatim* and Carl Rogers's *On Becoming a Person.*[33] Pop evangelical Christian psychology and pop secular psychology were amazingly similar in their message. Yet evangelical writers rarely acknowledged the similarity of their message to that of secular pop psychology. Rather, the emergence of the Christian counseling industry appeared to evangelical Christians as unique, a true Christian therapy for emotional ills, in contrast to secular therapies.

Early in my career I spoke at a number of Christian seminars on what I now view as pop psychology. I even tried to write some popular books. Yet these books never got past the manuscript phase. Christian publishing houses were not interested. In retrospect, I believe I could not fit my perspective into the Christian counseling industry perspective. For one, I was (and remain) not a particularly compelling popular writer. Second, I am too skeptical and too critical. On one occasion I sent out what I believed to be an excellent manuscript on the problem of pride among Christians entitled *Escape from Self.* Publisher after publisher returned the manuscript, explaining that their readers "did not want to read such a negative message." Thus ended my aspirations to join the ranks of popular Christian authors.

An examination of four successful authors—Bruce Larson, Tim LaHaye, David Seamands and Robert Schuller—provides poignant examples of Collins's characterization of popular Christian counselors. None of these authors are psychiatrists, nor do they profess psychiatric knowledge and skills, yet I believe their approach and popularity have significantly influenced many Christians who have entered psychiatric training during the past twenty-five years. The approach taken by many evangelical Christian psychiatrists in their practices has been shaped by these popular writers.

Bruce Larson is a Presbyterian minister who has become a popular writer in Christian counseling circles. In *Living on the Growing Edge* he summarizes his basic view: Jesus Christ is the Great Physician, and if we but obtain new insights into the teachings of Christ, we will be able to deal with the core human problems in the late twentieth century, such as the need for wholeness, the need for healing and the need to overcome fear. He suggests six steps to handle fear: analyze your fear; pay attention to healthy fears; don't fight unhealthy fears; learn to laugh at yourself; risk failure; and recognize fear as faith in reverse.[34] Larson calls extensively on the works of the Jewish psychiatrist Viktor Frankl in developing his practical counseling technique. Frankl wrote extensively about his experiences in a Nazi concentration camp and how they enabled him to find meaning in his life. His subsequent practice of psychiatry was devoted to helping his patients, in turn, to find meaning.[35]

Larson's basic approach to fears is that one should not attempt to escape or fight them; persons should recognize fears as friends that "keep us from destroying ourselves or others physically, mentally, emotionally and socially."[36] He uses the example of the fears learned by children who develop "a healthy respect for busy streets, hot stoves, and sharp knives."[37] In other words, Larson suggests that fear is not so bad. This approach, however, is in contrast to Frankl's approach to fear, for Frankl would never have suggested that the fears experienced by the Jews during World War II could be friends. Rather, Frankl describes how he coped, as best he could, with a pain and fear he never would wish on others. Fear was a reality to Frankl, but never a friend. Larson, on the other hand, suggests that if you can laugh at yourself, if you can risk failure and if you can learn to give yourself over to God, fear can be a friend as opposed to an enemy. Therefore if you are to "live on the growing edge," you must accept and welcome the emotion of fear. Larson basically describes a process of desensitizing oneself, a process well grounded in the behavioral and cognitive therapies of modern psychology and psychiatry. Yet he does not readily acknowledge the limits of such therapy.

For example, a woman from an evangelical Christian background in her mid-forties will not leave her house because of an unrealistic fear of contamination by bacteria. Her fear has isolated her from God and her friends. Psychiatrists recognize this woman as suffering from a phobic disorder with perhaps significant obsessive-compulsive traits. She is paralyzed by her fear, to the point that she has become virtually dysfunctional. How is she to accept Larson's message? His advice seems reasonable, but she cannot follow his six steps. A psychiatrist tells her that she needs to take a medication, perhaps Nardil, which will help her overcome her phobia. Taking a medication is far from living on the growing edge. If God has given her this fear in order to strengthen her faith, then she should attempt to overcome the phobia on her own.

The problem of severe phobic disorder could benefit from a conversation between psychiatrists and Christian theologians. If a woman experiencing a severe phobia would have difficulty negotiating a "cure," imagine the problems Barbara would face if she were to be asked to face her demons through Larson's six steps (see chapter one). Popular Christian writers, however, leave little room for such conversation and appear to have little interest in the severe problems that extend beyond the ordinary fears of everyday life. They may refer the severe phobic to a professional counselor, but once that person is out of sight, she or he is out of mind.

Tim LaHaye's approach to emotional problems comes from a perspective that differs from Larson's. He attacks one of the most severe emotional problems experienced by humankind—major depression. In the preface to his book *How to Win over Depression,* LaHaye describes his own experience with the illness: "I experienced the most devastating event of my life since my father died. Struck by my first serious wave of depression, I could for the first time truly identify with the cold, apathetic, hopeless feeling of the depressed."[38]

His recovery encouraged him to write a book that sold over a half-million copies. LaHaye's goal was to "help many others realize the true cause of a major emotional culprit and offer a workable remedy."[39] He then prescribes a treatment guaranteed to succeed: "Of one thing I am confident: you do not have to be depressed. . . . I'm convinced that by using the formula in this book, you can avoid ever being depressed again."[40]

LaHaye bases his formula on the work of Aaron Beck (see chapter three)—that is, he proposes a spiritual version of cognitive therapy for depression. LaHaye appeals to evangelical Christians by sprinkling biblical quotes liberally throughout his writing. Among the "ten steps to victory over depression" he includes the following:

☐ accept Jesus Christ as your Savior

☐ walk in the Spirit

☐ forgive those who sin against you

☐ practice creative imagery daily through prayer

In other words, LaHaye intermixes the inspirational message of the evangelical minister with the practical message of the cognitive therapist. Yet he scarcely attempts to reconcile, much less integrate, the two approaches. After grounding his steps to victory over depression in acceptance of Jesus and dependence on him, his formula encourages the power-of-positive-thinking, mind-over-matter approach of the cognitive therapies, along with a scattering of the imagery therapy used by behavioral therapists such as the psychiatrist Joseph Wolpe (see below). For example, the reader is encouraged to fashion a new image of self through a daily prayer/imagination exercise: "accept yourself as a creature of God; accept God's forgiveness for sins; . . . visualize yourself as God is shaping you; always be positive."[41] Combined with appropriate medical therapies, according to LaHaye, these practical steps assure the reader that depression will never be a problem again.

Depression is a chronic illness. Some lives are plagued by chronic stress, loss and disappointments such that it is extremely difficult, if not impossible, to maintain a positive attitude. Jeremiah, the weeping prophet, witnessed the destruction of Jerusalem and went through one insult and torment after another. He finally expressed the extent of his depression in his Lamentations. In this book, included in both the Jewish and the Christian canon, Jeremiah expresses virtually no hope for himself or his people. Trust in the Lord for Jeremiah was not analogous to positive thinking:

I am the man who has seen affliction
   by the rod of his wrath.
He has driven me away and made me walk
   in darkness rather than light. . . .
Even when I call out or cry for help,
   he shuts out my prayer. . . .
He pierced my heart with arrows from his quiver. . . .
He has filled me with bitter herbs
   and sated me with gall. (Lam 3:1-15)

The scriptural basis of LaHaye's approach to depression is therefore questionable. Though he quotes Scripture frequently, he usually extracts passages to support his formula, as opposed to searching the Scriptures themselves for a deeper understanding of the pain of depression. The ancient biblical writings are filled with wisdom relevant to the depressed in the twentieth century. The ancient writers both expressed and empathized with persons suffering emotional pain. No formulas were provided to guarantee freedom from depression.

Some persons experiencing depression may improve with the aid of popular Christian counseling. Others recover with the use of secular psychotherapies. The most severe may recover only with the use of medication. Still others recover from depression spontaneously. Unfortunately, if a person such as Jason (chapter one) experiences a severe depression, regardless of the therapy used, recovery is not assured, and if recovery occurs the likelihood of relapse into depression in the future is high, probably greater than 50 percent.

A conversation between popular writers, such as LaHaye, and psychiatrists about the realities of severe depression could be beneficial to both. The popularity of LaHaye's writings suggests that he is speaking a language understood by many persons suffering from depression, a language of hope from which psychiatry could learn. On the other hand, LaHaye and other popular Christian writers must recognize the chronic nature of the disorders that they too easily suggest are totally preventable.

David Seamands is yet another popular writer within the evangelical Christian counseling community. He served as a pastor for the United Methodist Church as well as a counselor to staff and students at Asbury College and Asbury Theological Seminary in Kentucky. Like Larson and LaHaye, Seamands came from a seminary background but ventured into the field of counseling because he perceived that the regular ministries of the church were not correcting the problems he felt were pervasive among the people with whom he interacted.

I was failing to help two groups of people through the regular ministries of the church. Their problems were not being solved by the preaching of the word. . . . One group [was] driven into futility and loss of confidence in God's power . . . while they kept up the outward observances of praying

and professing. . . . The other [was] moving toward phoniness . . .
repressing their inner feelings and denying to themselves that anything
was seriously wrong.[42]

Seamands focused his new ministry on what he called "special care and
prayer for damaged emotions and unhealed memories." More than Larson
and LaHaye, Seamands uses imagery in healing the emotions.

Seamands's approach is to take his counselees on a journey into the past,
a journey not parallel to that of psychoanalysis. He emphasizes reinterpret-
ing the past in the light of God's grace and love. For example, Seamands
describes a counselee who suffered from a poor self-image that derived in
large part from her father's view of her as an unattractive young woman.[43]
Her father would say to her, "You know, you just can't make a peach out of
a potato." The young woman came to feel more and more like an ugly potato.
Seamands's therapeutic approach was to reprogram her self-image. "We
had to walk through those painful memories with our Lord, turning them
over to him for healing. I often called her 'God's peach' or 'my peach.' "[44]

The approach to therapy taken by Seamands derives from behavioral
therapies developed during the 1950s by psychiatrist Joseph Wolpe.[45] If a
patient experienced severe anxiety related to a stimulus, such as fear of
closed-in places, Wolpe prescribed teaching him or her to visualize the
stimulus, perhaps a closed place, while practicing relaxation. The stimulus
would thus lose its potential to create anxiety, for relaxation is incompatible
with anxiety. To induce relaxation, Wolpe encouraged relaxing specific
muscle groups while imagining a peaceful experience, such as reclining in
a lounge chair on the beach. Seamands therefore has put a spiritual spin on
the behavioral therapy technique of reciprocal inhibition.

Seamands's approach to healing is almost identical to that of Bernie S.
Siegel. Siegel, a surgeon in New Haven, Connecticut, published a popular
book, *Love, Medicine and Miracles,* in 1986.[46] Here he surveys a rather
substantial body of scientific literature suggesting that positive thinking
decreases anger and that love actualized through imaging is associated with
good health outcomes. "The mind's power is available to us all the time."[47]
For example, he describes a man with a cancer that had spread to his brain.
Under hypnosis, this man imagined that he entered a room within his brain

that controlled blood supply. He was instructed to turn off the valve that controlled the blood flow to his tumor.[48] The tumor subsequently shrank to one-fourth its original size.

This type of healing is not generally accepted by modern technological society. There is growing interest, however, in the efficacy of the intangibles of healing among physicians as well as Christian counselors. Siegel has received wide acceptance by the public. The similarities between his imaging techniques and underlying theories and those of Seamands are striking, so Seamands's approach is not uniquely Christian.

Though Seamands's approach is not unique, he has found a most receptive audience to his writings and seminars. First, he provides evangelicals hope beyond traditional psychiatry: the hope of healing through the miracle of the grace of God. Second, he appeals to grace, especially the role of Jesus Christ, in the healing process. In this way he is unlike Christian counselors such as LaHaye who emphasize practical Christian wisdom. Third, Seamands cuts against the grain of traditional counseling, for he provides personal testimony that his former traditional approach was ineffective and his new approach provides a much-needed alternative. Finally, Seamands has little formal training in psychiatry or psychology, a fact that enhances his credibility among some Christians as he expounds his apparently unique therapeutic approach.

The effectiveness of Seamands's approach is not at issue. It has not been proved either more or less effective than traditional therapies. It is rather more important to recognize that his therapy is borrowed from secular medicine and psychiatry, mixed with Christian symbols and packaged as a unique therapy for evangelical Christians.

No discussion of the popularization of Christian counseling is complete without mention of the myriad self-help books that have been published in recent years which straddle the boundary between healing emotional problems and providing guidance for everyday living. A good example of a popular minister at this boundary is Robert Schuller. In the introduction to his book *Tough Times Never Last, but Tough People Do!* Schuller encourages his reader to "take action to make a bold and daring move . . . make a creative transition. This book will get you started on the path to success once again."[49]

Schuller comes from the tradition of Norman Vincent Peale and is not clearly associated with the evangelical tradition. Yet his writings have been popular among evangelicals. *Tough Times Never Last* is directed not to the emotionally disturbed but to ordinary people who seek motivation to get their lives going. Schuller believes that everyone has problems, whether physical, emotional or social. Success depends not on whether individuals have problems but on whether they are tough enough to survive the problems.

He suggests six principles that pertain to all problems: every living human being has problems; every problem has a limited life span; every problem holds positive possibilities; every problem will change you; you can choose how your problem will change you; and there is a negative and positive choice associated with every problem. Explicit in these steps is that one not only will come out tough but will come out a winner, as expressed in the aphorisms scattered through the book—for example, "You won't win if you don't begin" and "The me I see. . . is the me I'll be."

In a competitive, aggressive and entrepreneurial society, Schuller has great appeal. He emphasizes success, the cornerstone of the American way of life. His simple, practical approach can be grasped by virtually anyone who reads his writings. He is an excellent communicator and has magnetic personal appeal. Though Schuller does not profess to be a counselor or an evangelical, many Christian counselors choose to model themselves after him rather than to practice traditional counseling. A well-known evangelical counselor once told me, "I'm going to give up my counseling practice. I believe I can help more persons with a positive and popular message delivered through seminars and written in books than I can by working one on one with individuals."

Yet Schuller represents a trend that could undermine the healing of Christians who are experiencing severe emotional suffering. Counselors treating such persons simply cannot follow Schuller's exhortations. Every positive exhortation will be met initially by an equally negative response. People suffering severe emotional suffering can easily wear down the counselor who offers a single, simple prescription for healing. The counselee keeps coming back to the counselor with the message "I tried what you said, but it doesn't work." After one or two sessions of positive, upbeat exhortation, counselor and counselee both become discouraged. The relationship often ends in frustration for both parties.

It is easier to write books and hold seminars where the encounter is brief and upbeat than it is to work day in and day out with someone suffering a chronic and serious mental illness. Christian counselors who wish to make a name for themselves as popular writers and speakers have therefore shown little inclination to deal with the most severe emotional problems. This is not surprising. One does not attain popularity by speaking to a relatively small percentage of the population, a percentage that will not respond to a good book or seminar.

The trend to popularize Christian counseling has left little room for meaningful conversation with psychiatry. The popular writer is more interested in borrowing from psychiatry what might be useful as a practical guide to living than in forming partnerships for treating the most difficult problems. Popular counselors are more inclined to deliver their message to large groups than in ongoing one-on-one relationships. They are more interested in prescriptive answers to prototypical problems than in iterative interactions over time with the unique life history of a person suffering severe emotional pain. These popular counselors are, I believe, well-meaning and receive considerable feedback that their efforts are successful, much more than the typical pastoral counselor or psychiatrist. I believe their greatest failing is that they have become satisfied with their prescriptive answers. They no longer ask the tough questions.

The Professionalization of Christian Counseling

During the late 1960s and early 1970s, at the same time that some evangelical pastors were popularizing Christian counseling, a number of young women and men from evangelical backgrounds entered psychiatric and clinical psychological training. Fuller Theological Seminary in Pasadena, California, had been founded by evangelicals in 1947. The Fuller School of Psychology admitted its first class in 1965.[50] John Finch, a practicing psychologist, was a major influence in founding the school. He was especially concerned with the philosophical issues that underlie the tensions between Christian and contemporary psychological worldviews. Unlike pastoral counselors from mainline Protestant Christian churches, Finch was a professional psychologist with a strong evangelical background.[51] In his dissertation he suggested that an alternative worldview to that of Freud, a view that incorporates the spiritual, should undergird counseling. In many ways the school was established to provide an alternative rather than a complement to Freudian psychotherapy.

The School of Psychology at Fuller, nevertheless, worked hard to demonstrate to the secular community that its program was legitimate and deserved the respect of secular psychologists. The first dean selected was Lee Edward Travis, a respected academic psychologist known for his work in electroencephalography and speech pathology.[52] Travis had undergone a profound religious experience (an evangelical-like conversion) and had a sense of the emptiness resulting from human attempts to gain control over the human condition. Yet integrating psychology and Christianity proved difficult at Fuller. Some professionals viewed psychology as an autonomous science into which it would be presumptuous to introduce evangelical theology. Others sought to discover and teach the advantage of Christian counseling over secular counseling. Travis clearly fell into the former category.

As dean, he worked diligently to ensure that the program excelled according to the conventional standards of clinical psychology. Only then could the faculty expand its energies to the difficult problems of theological integration and debate.[53] This eventually led to the accreditation of the clinical psychology program by the American Psychological Association in 1974. Today the school houses one of the largest accredited clinical psychology training programs in the United States. The school provides a comfortable environment for evangelical Christians to obtain excellent professional training. Fuller has produced a cadre of professional psychologists with a strong commitment to the Christian faith. The integrative task, however, continues to prove difficult.

Fuller was by no means the only evangelical institution to be attracted to psychology. Biola University is a large evangelical school with a sizable seminary which also has a school of psychology, the Rosemead Graduate

School of Professional Psychology, in La Mirada, California. Many, if not most, seminaries have departments of psychology and pastoral counseling. The programs at these schools range from the academic to a practical, nonscholarly approach to counseling. Many of the professors who teach in these programs make attempts at integration but find accommodation a much easier task. They have therefore uncritically incorporated an entire range of therapeutic methods of counseling into their training programs—methods ranging from hypnosis to behavior therapy.

A movement simultaneously began in psychiatry but was much less widespread and less institutionalized. The Christian psychiatry movement began at Duke University under the direction of William Wilson during the early 1970s and was continued at the University of Georgia under the direction of Mansell Pattison during the late 1970s and early 1980s. These psychiatrists established training programs to produce a distinctive group of psychiatrists, so-called Christian psychiatrists. Christian psychiatry as a movement did not include everyone professing a Christian faith and practicing psychiatry. Instead it attracted medical school graduates with an evangelical background. I was attracted to Duke for psychiatric training because I could receive supervision from Bill Wilson, an evangelical Christian who was a respected academic psychiatrist at an outstanding medical center.

Neither Wilson nor Pattison became especially well known for their popular writings, yet both were well regarded among professional colleagues. Each had achieved considerable status within the ranks of psychiatry prior to their efforts to express their Christian beliefs more openly. Before the movement begun by Wilson, psychiatrists from evangelical backgrounds were isolated and, like popular Christian counselors, attracted attention among evangelicals, not psychiatrists, if they attracted attention at all. Wilson, in contrast, attracted significant attention among his psychiatric colleagues both locally and regionally.

Bill Wilson tells his story in *The Grace to Grow.*[54] He was a respected neuropsychiatrist specializing in electroencephalography at the time when Freudian psychiatry dominated American psychiatry. In 1965 he underwent a dramatic conversion to Christianity and became a vocal and aggressive spokesperson for evangelical Christianity. Wilson's willingness to step out, speak for Christianity and explore the interface between psychiatry and religion with no fear that his faith would be undermined was a powerful example to those who sought training with him. Seniority as a psychiatrist and tenure in the medical school helped to secure his ability to challenge the basic assumptions of mainstream psychiatry. He encouraged the young Christians who came to Duke for psychiatric training to pursue academic careers and seriously address the tough questions that would emerge during their training. Persons trained by Wilson are currently on faculty at many psychiatric training programs throughout the United States, including Duke, the Menninger Clinic, Loma Linda School of Medicine, Michigan State University School of Medicine, Bowman Gray School of Medicine and the Unified Armed Services School of Medicine.

E. Mansel Pattison had an equally strong, but not as aggressive, desire to incorporate the Christian faith into psychiatry. He was an established academic psychiatrist when he accepted the chair in psychiatry at the University of Georgia School of Medicine in the late 1970s. Though Pattison was more mainline Protestant in his beliefs, he recruited to his department a core of evangelical Christian faculty members, many of whom had trained at Duke under Wilson. With this nucleus of Christian faculty, he established a program that attracted additional men and women to psychiatry from the ranks of evangelical Christians.

Pattison originally addressed the interface between psychiatry and religion as did persons like Karl Menninger and Gregory Zilboorg. That is, he began to ask questions about religion as it related to psychiatry from the perspective of the psychiatrist. For example, in a 1966 article he explored four ideological positions regarding psychotherapy:

☐ reductionists, psychiatrists who view mental health as solely a question of scientific psychology or entirely a religious issue, respectively

☐ dualists, who believe in two domains and that one qualified therapist can be effective in both

☐ alternativists, who view the problem as usually psychological but believe that either the minister or the psychotherapist can fulfill the therapeutic task

☐ specialists, who maintain two separate tasks, requiring both mental health professional and pastor[55]

At that time Pattison did not favor one position over another, but later he became a dualist (in his terms), attempting to train persons in both the Christian faith and psychiatry so that qualified Christian psychiatrists could treat the psychiatric and the spiritual. Pattison did not experience a dramatic conversion as did Wilson, yet he was anchored firmly in his faith during the later years of his life, and his theories of psychiatry progressively derived more from his faith.

The Christian psychiatry movement has not developed as extensively as the movement in psychology, yet it has been a relatively strong one. In 1985 approximately one hundred psychiatrists belonged to the psychiatry section of the Christian Medical Society, a society devoted to supporting Christians of predominantly evangelical faith in the practice of medicine.[56] The psychiatry section regularly attracts seventy-five to one hundred psychiatrists to events associated with the annual meeting of the American Psychiatric Association.

Even as young evangelical Christians were seeking training in psychiatry during the 1970s and 1980s, more senior psychiatrists were affirming their faith and its relevance to their practice, thus attaching themselves to the movement. Some, like Bill Wilson, underwent dramatic conversions. Others experienced more gradual but substantive changes in their views of psychiatry and began to incorporate their faith more thoroughly into their practice. The movement attracted persons from both evangelical and nonevangelical backgrounds and perspectives, yet it tended to be dominated by evangelicals.

Before 1970 psychiatrists who openly professed Christian faith were rare, despite extensive literature on the relation of psychiatry/psychology and religion.[57] Those who did express their beliefs and attempted to incorporate them into their practices generally underwent conversion to Christianity, or at least a reaffirmation of their faith, after they had completed psychiatric training and were well established in practice or in an academic career. Only after 1970 did Christians, especially from evangelical backgrounds, seek training in psychiatry in substantial numbers because they viewed psychiatry as a means by which they could express their ministry. The Freudian barrier to Christians' entering psychiatry had been broken.

The Christian psychiatry movement, however, has now lost much of the identity and momentum it achieved during the 1970s. I suspect one reason is that the battle many evangelicals felt they would have to fight as psychiatrists never materialized, although this threat of battle led evangelicals to firmly establish themselves in their faith tradition and struggle with anti-Christian theories of human nature. In other words, the need for a Christian psychiatry movement dissipated because after a few years of struggle most secular psychiatrists were not concerned that evangelical Christians sought psychiatric training. As many evangelical Christians are today seeking training in psychiatry as during the 1970s, but they do not identify themselves as part of a distinct movement, do not seek a program of training that emphasizes Christian psychiatry (with few exceptions) and rarely feel isolated from or in serious conflict with their non-Christian colleagues.

This does not mean that psychiatrists with roots in Christianity do not meet together and discuss goals and concerns regarding the practice of their profession within the context of their faith. Neither does it mean that Christian psychiatrists no longer view themselves as working in uncharted territory which would force them to reflect on their practice activities as well as their beliefs. What has disappeared is the "we versus they" attitude that placed evangelical Christians and psychoanalysts in direct confrontation.

The Christian psychiatry movement grew out of the evangelical tradition, not the tradition of pastoral care. Little emphasis has been placed on exposing religious beliefs to psychiatric explorations. Rather, Christian psychiatrists have been reshaping their practice of psychiatry to incorporate the principles of Christian salvation and healing. Psychiatry, as a profession, is the vehicle by which these evangelicals work to serve members of the Christian community and provide answers to persons outside the Christian community who have unsuccessfully sought relief from emotional suffering through traditional therapies.

Evangelism, as well as therapy, was a goal of the Christian psychiatry movement. Prayer, Bible study and participation in a Christian community were ingredients in Christian psychotherapy. Wilson expresses this view as follows:

While Christian psychotherapy employs many of the same techniques used in secular psychotherapy, it has as its primary goal for the patient, his or her reconciliation with God through faith in Christ. . . . Through conversion, a patient receives God's in-dwelling Holy Spirit—a very personal counselor, comforter, and source of healing power. In addition, he is also given the potential for no less than an entirely new personality. Drawing upon this transforming and healing power of the Holy Spirit, the Christian psychotherapist works to cleanse his or her patients of painful emotions and undesirable behavior. He has at his employ a wide variety of therapeutic methods and techniques, including such particular Christian tools as conversion, prayer, forgiveness, and the Eucharist. He encourages in his or her patients the adoption of new behavior and values, biblically based, that will serve to make a favorable difference in the patient's life.[58]

The role of evangelism in the practice of psychiatry has been hotly debated, even among evangelical psychiatrists. Psychiatrists from other faith traditions have viewed it as unprofessional, if not unethical, and significant tension has arisen when evangelistic Christian psychiatrists practiced alongside more traditional secular colleagues. Yet the issue has generated much more heat than light. Honest, open discussion of the ethical implications of Christian psychotherapy, as described by Wilson above, has rarely materialized across faith traditions.

Having found myself in the middle of a tense atmosphere at Duke during the late 1970s and early 1980s, I am intimately acquainted with the tension. On one hand, I recognized the potential for coercion, since psychiatrists have significant authority in their relationships with people who are vulnerable and seeking help. Yet at the core of the evangelical tradition is evangelism, spreading the good news of Jesus Christ to those in distress. Like most of my evangelical colleagues, I never actually resolved the conflict. The choice before us seemed either to become openly evangelistic in our practice or to follow a more traditional approach of therapy. I opted for the latter approach, though I cannot articulate a reason for my decision with which I truly feel comfortable. I am more comfortable, however, than I was in the tense atmosphere created by the evangelism-in-psychotherapy controversy.

What I (along with my Christian and non-Christian colleagues) lost following the conflict was an opportunity to address basic issues, values, culture and the philosophical implications that underlie traditional psycho-therapies. The conflict tended to polarize evangelical Christians and other psychiatrists who were practicing side by side. Then we found a language and topic about which we could agree: neuropsychiatry. Friendly dialogue was once again established.

This view, granted, is personal and biased. My colleagues may evaluate the relationship between evangelical Christian psychiatrists and their col-leagues from other faith traditions very differently. I do know, however, that the tension, at least at Duke, had disappeared for all practical purposes by the latter 1980s. As the tension disappeared, so did the conversation.

The original strongholds of training in evangelical Christian psychiatry no longer remain strongholds. Wilson left Duke during the 1980s, and after his departure the program in Christian psychiatry evaporated. Pattison was fatally injured in an automobile accident in the late 1980s. Following his death, most of the faculty at the University of Georgia who had been attracted there by the Christian perspective went elsewhere. A program in Christian psychiatry has continued in at least two institutions, both of which derive from more mainline Christian traditions and therefore are natural settings for Christians who practice psychiatry.

Pine Rest Hospital in Grand Rapids, Michigan, is an established, free-standing psychiatric institution operated by the Christian Reformed Church. It is staffed predominantly by Christians and has continued a strong program of integrating Christian faith and the practice of psychiatry. Though adver-tised as a Christian hospital, the institution does not advocate a unique Christian psychiatry but a Christian mission in the practice of psychiatry. The hospital served as a training site for psychiatric residents from Michi-gan State School of Medicine for many years.

Loma Linda University School of Medicine in California, established by the Seventh-day Adventists, maintains a department of psychiatry that emphasizes the integration of Christianity and psychiatry. Seminars in psychiatry and religion (with an emphasis on Christianity) continue in training programs such as Menninger's and Harvard. Otherwise the remnants of the Christian psychiatry movement have diverged from mainstream psychiatry and dissociated themselves from academic institutions.

The Christian psychiatry movement, however, is not dead. It has become institutionalized outside mainstream psychiatry but, interestingly, has developed a rapprochement of sorts with mainstream psychiatry. During the early and middle 1980s a number of psychiatric hospitals, or psychiatric units within general hospitals, developed special Christian therapy units. Initially these units were established by psychiatrists who had been trained at institutions such as Duke and the University of Georgia and who negotiated with hospital administrators to develop special units for Christian therapy. Though tension often arose between the directors of these units and other psychiatrists within the hospital, hospital administrators saw the benefits of the units as greater than the risks. Specifically, at a time when filling beds was becoming a problem for hospitals, the attraction of Christian patients to a facility—Christians who are usually good about paying their bills and who perhaps would not have sought psychiatric care otherwise—was viewed as a special advantage. In addition, some hospital administrators recognized the potential problems evangelical Christians might experience with mainstream psychiatry. Many of these hospitals served communities where a significant minority, if not a majority, of their clientele were from an evangelical Christian background. Administrators were therefore sympathetic to the perceived need for psychiatric treatment programs with an evangelical orientation.

The next step in the Christian psychiatry movement was the development of a network of these Christian psychiatry units, providing an identity for these units nationwide. The networks include Kairos (launched by one of the nation's leading providers of psychiatric services), Rapha and New Life Treatment Centers. The Minirth-Meier New Life Treatment Centers have become popular in recent years and serve as an illustration of the Christian psychiatry industry during the late twentieth century. Frank Minirth and Paul Meier trained in psychiatry at the University of Arkansas. Following their training they worked briefly with theological seminaries and later formed an independent counseling center in Fort Worth, Texas. Together and separately they have written popular Christian counseling books similar to those of LaHaye, Seamands and Larson. It is the marketing of Christian psychiatry, however, that sets them apart from Wilson and Pattison.

Name recognition from their writings, as well as radio and television appearances on syndicated Christian programs, has allowed Minirth and Meier to establish a network of treatment centers in many parts of the United States. Brochures for these centers advertise treatment for a variety of problems, such as depression, stress, panic attacks, phobias, codependency/dependency, chemical dependency, compulsive sexual behavior, compulsive eating disorders and problems of adolescence. They speak specifically to evangelical Christians:

> We can help you or a loved one. We are a place you can trust. . . . The primary goal of our program is to create a warm, integrative and non-threatening therapeutic environment, where people can work through and resolve their conflicts with respect to their values and beliefs. . . . We are firmly committed to a personal faith in Jesus Christ, and emphasize consistent use of God's word as the primary resource of strength and understanding. This belief is combined with the highest quality clinical care available in proven twelve-step principles of recovery.[59]

The New Life Centers provide a statement of faith for those who wish to test the Christian orientation of their treatment programs. This statement affirms the inspiration and authority of the Scriptures and the Holy Spirit's power of regeneration. Services offered include psychotherapy, medication management, consultation and evaluation, educational seminars, and promised close cooperation with local churches and pastors.

Free-standing psychiatric hospitals and hospital-based psychiatric programs have accepted programs such as the New Life Centers with amazing ease. The acceptance of such a program on a psychiatry unit in a general hospital would have been unheard of twenty-five years ago. What has changed?

Economics undoubtedly have played a major role, but not the only role. Psychiatry has become much less dogmatic in its theories and therefore much more accommodating to persons of all faith persuasions. Perhaps this is a natural response to an increasingly diverse society. Similar programs could as easily be established to meet the needs of countless other faith traditions if it were determined that special programs were needed or would be accepted by that community of believers, would provide a standard of care to which all psychiatrists are held, and would attract patients to treatment centers. The New Life Centers meet these criteria and therefore have been well accepted by some—and reluctantly accepted by most— mental health professionals working in the hospitals where the centers have been established. The New Life program has matured into a packaged, well-marketed and attractive promise of hope to evangelical Christians suffering from emotional problems.

Psychiatrists working with these centers have not, in large part, remained attached to mainstream psychiatry, as would be evidenced by active participation in the American Psychiatric Association and the American College of Psychiatry. The psychiatrists practicing in these units have sought their professional colleagues among other Christian counselors (with whom they work closely) and have developed social networks within the evangelical community. Therefore these programs are parallel to, but interact little with, mainstream psychiatry.

The effectiveness of these programs has yet to be determined. I suspect that the overall success rate is no better and no worse than for general psychiatric units and that these centers "feel right" to many evangelicals who suffer emotional problems but fear exposing their innermost thoughts to a person from a different faith. For problems such as chemical dependency, these programs may be especially effective; they provide something recognized by virtually all as useful in overcoming chemical dependency, a strong religious motivation and the support of a group of common believers. For example, the twelve steps of Alcoholics Anonymous are easily integrated into Christian psychiatry programs. In their brochure the New Life Centers promise a professional group "dedicated to integrating Biblical principles with clinical principles and proven twelve-step principles," the very twelve steps of Alcoholic Anonymous.

Questions have been raised, however, even among evangelicals, about this "franchising of hope." These programs are for profit and promote their services on Christian radio stations and in Christian literature. If a person's insurance won't pay, he or she is not likely to be admitted. Christian charity plays little role in these units. The units have been criticized for marketing their psychiatry as unique when in actuality there is no coherent form of practice that renders the psychiatry they practice any different from current secular psychiatry, except for the use of Christian symbols, language and rituals.[60] Yet the health care system today is rapidly changing and is marketed via symbols intended to attract a clientele, so marketing with the use of attractive symbols is not unique to Christian psychiatry.

The units have also been criticized for blurring the boundaries between therapy and evangelism and thereby possibly undermining the authority of the church. In other words, these units potentially can become alternatives to the church as support networks for persons suffering emotionally, especially if their outpatient and chronic-care programs expand. In the final analysis, however, the success or failure of these units will be their financial viability. If they are accepted by Christians and prove financially valuable to hospitals, theoretical concerns about them will have little influence.

The Politicization of Christian Counseling

Despite bestselling popular Christian counseling books, despite well-attended Christian counseling seminars, despite the influx of evangelical Christians into psychiatry and other mental health professions, Christian counseling has not established a distinctive niche in mental health services. Popular self-help books mostly are applied secular psychiatry and psychology adapted to an evangelical orientation. The evangelicals who now enter psychiatry usually practice modern psychiatry with some incorporation of Christian principles. Coupled with the supportive evangelical community, persons with credentials in psychiatry, psychology and other mental health disciplines have been successful in establishing their practices but not necessarily successful in the difficult task of integration. As pastoral counseling incorporated Rogerian therapy virtually unchanged during the mid-twentieth century, the Christian counseling industry has incorporated neuropsychiatry and cognitive therapy. Christian counseling and Christian psychiatry have failed to establish a clearly unique or superior package of mental health services.

In a progressively market-oriented health services environment, persons suffering from emotional problems can choose from a smorgasbord of therapies ranging from self-help groups to medications prescribed by a physician. In what way could evangelical Christian counselors assert their distinctive identity? Many Christians in the evangelical tradition as well as many pastoral counselors have focused on marriage and family therapy, and this has become their niche. Such a focus, in my opinion, is natural and potentially most productive. In what better way could the evangelical community explore severe emotional suffering in its social and cultural context than to explore the impact of such suffering on families? How better could the evangelical community understand the impact of dysfunctional relationships on persons than by exploring dysfunctional families? What better model could be found for understanding the potential of the faith community to become a healing community than the model of a functional family? Yet evangelical marriage and family therapists pursued a different strategy.

From a focus on marriage and the family, Christian counselors have gravitated to the political arena and have become among the strongest proponents of "family values" and the Christian right. Of course evangelical Christians are not unique in moving concern about emotional suffering to the political arena. The gay rights movement has politicized the emotional experience of persons who experience homosexual desires but feel constrained and conflicted in expressing these desires. Feminists certainly moved the emotional and moral conflict regarding abortion to the political arena with political rhetoric such as "a woman's right to choose." Relevant to this discussion, however, is that evangelical Christians have been equally willing and aggressive in moving "family values" issues to the political arena.

Marriage and family therapy was at one time the province of secular psychiatry and psychology. The golden age of family therapy extended from approximately 1950 to 1975 in the United States.[61] Though its roots stretched back to the late 1940s, significant leaders in marriage and family therapy arose during the 1950s. Nathan Ackerman, the best known of the early family therapists, advocated a focus on family from the perspective of a child psychiatrist firmly grounded in psychoanalytic therapy. He recognized that

> none of us live our lives utterly alone. Those who try are doomed to a miserable existence. It can fairly be said that some aspects of life experience are more individual than social, and others more social than individual. Nevertheless, principally we live with others, and in early years almost exclusively with members of our own family.[62]

Many and varied disciplines informed family therapy. Gregory Bateson, firmly grounded in anthropology, identified communication problems in families, specifically describing the double-bind hypothesis of schizophrenia. He, along with his colleagues, hypothesized that a major contributor to schizophrenia in children was an ambivalent message of a mother, verbally expressing that she loved the child but physically withdrawing that love. This places the child in an ongoing double bind that was theorized to precipitate schizophrenia (a hypothesis that has been largely abandoned today). Other psychiatrists, such as Lyman Wynne, applied theories of group dynamics to family therapy and encouraged the therapist to assume an observer position and to clarify the process of family interactions. These investigator/therapists produced a remarkably rich literature on marriage and family therapy through the 1960s and 1970s.

The rise of neuropsychiatry coupled with the unwillingness of insurance companies to pay for family therapy forced psychiatry to abandoned both the study of the family and the practice of family therapy by the mid-1980s. Social workers and psychologists provided family therapy as an adjunct to the medication and individual psychotherapy administered by psychiatrists, usually within the context of a comprehensive mental health plan. Family therapy moved to the periphery as the patient in the context of a sociocultural environment became less important as a theoretical basis in the practice of psychiatry.

At the very time psychiatrists were abandoning marriage and family therapy, evangelical Christian counselors, among others, recognized the vacuum and found their niche in the mental health service system, a niche where they could excel and which was compatible with evangelical Christian values. By far the best example of the movement to marriage and family therapy by a Christian counselor is James C. Dobson.

Dobson was a clinical professor of pediatrics (psychology) at the University of Southern California School of Medicine. He also served as a school psychologist and observed the problems children encountered with their families firsthand. In 1970 he published a book, *Dare to Discipline.*[63] Three circumstances surrounding this book are noteworthy.

First, it was published by an evangelical publishing house, Tyndale, as opposed to a publisher that typically published psychological works for the public at large. Just a few years prior Avon Books had published Haim Ginott's *Between Parent and Child,* a book that sold well over a million copies.[64] Interest in families was increasing, and Dobson recognized an untapped audience among evangelical Christians.

Second, Dobson took an approach to working with children most appealing to evangelical Christians, for it paralleled the approach to child rearing reflected in the biblical dictum "spare the rod and spoil the child" (see Prov 13:24). His goal was to provide a model of discipline that would lead to the raising of obedient, respectful children: "In a day of widespread drug usage, immorality, civil disobedience, vandalism, and violence, we must not depend on hope and luck to fashion the critical attitudes we value in our children. . . . Permissiveness has not just been a failure; it has been a disaster!"[65] He took the side of those "parents and teachers who believed in moral decency and wanted to instill responsible sexual attitudes in their children."[66]

Third, more than one million copies of *Dare to Discipline* had sold by 1983, firmly establishing Dobson as the leading spokesperson for the family among evangelical Christians. Dobson has published many books since, established a syndicated radio program that is carried by hundreds of radio stations throughout the United States—*Focus on the Family*—and developed an organization by the same name which is currently a multimillion-dollar enterprise. He has moved away from his academic roots and situated his operation on a free-standing campus in Colorado Springs, Colorado. Dobson has maintained little contact with secular professional organizations. Rather, he has entered the political arena. He has taken on numerous causes, virtually all of which focus on external "threats" to the family in our society. These include pornography, homosexuality, abortion and the elimination of prayer in schools.

The leap from marriage and family therapy to political action is not a long one. Many Americans believe that the family is under attack today. The culprits range from poverty to changing societal attitudes. The evangelical Christian marriage and family movement has taken the anxieties of persons about the family and translated them into fears of social and political forces that challenge traditional family values. These family values are equated with evangelical Christian values. Dobson has announced, "We are in a civil war of values and the prize to the victor is the next generation—our children and grandchildren."[67] The war is fought on a few key battlegrounds: abortion, which is perceived to render sexual intercourse out of wedlock acceptable; homosexuality, which supports an alternate lifestyle to the traditional family; pornography, which encourages sexual activities that extend beyond the bounds of Christian family values; and the abolition of prayer in schools, which emphasizes that school is not an extension of the Christian family.

Evangelical Christians, as a result of their concern about societal values, have developed a counterculture. Christian schools, established as an alternative to public education, emphasize family values, actively seek children from traditional families and intermix religious and secular instruction. Other evangelical Christians are electing to school their children at home. Reading materials, videotapes, movies and television programs suitable for family-oriented Christians are increasing in popularity. Christian television networks and family-oriented channels are now available to most subscribers of cable television. Family-oriented vacation sites and activities are widely marketed.

Yet evangelical Christians are making their greatest impact in local political elections. Though the Moral Majority of Jerry Falwell is no longer as visible as it was in the 1980s, evangelicals are a formidable political force today, as evidenced by the political revolution of November 1994. That political force is fueled by concern for family values.

This emphasis on political action and a Christian counterculture does not encourage conversation between psychiatrists and evangelical Christians. The focus on externals and on political action is accompanied by a deemphasis on understanding the internal struggles of the emotionally suffering and by attacks on nontraditional families. Though evangelical groups have developed singles ministries, ministries to single parents, ministries to older adults, inner-city ministries and ministries to the homeless, they have not incorporated these diverse groups into the church family. The message to the single young adult is to get married. The message to the divorced or widowed is, at least implicitly, to remarry. The evangelical church does not accept the apostle Paul's statement "Now to the unmarried and the widows I say: It is good for them to stay unmarried, as I am" (see 1 Cor 7:8, 10-11, 17).

Political attacks by evangelical Christians from a counseling platform have been primarily directed toward elected officials, not psychiatry. Nevertheless, conflict that derives in large part from the political concern of evangelicals is emerging within psychiatry on at least two fronts. First, a minority of psychiatrists, including many evangelicals, have attacked the prochoice position taken by the American Psychiatric Association (APA) on abortion. American Psychiatrists for Neutrality on Abortion have challenged the position of the APA and issued a position statement at the 1993 meeting of the American Psychiatric Association in San Francisco. The group does not wish the APA to take a prolife position, but rather to take no position in the abortion debate.

A second political conflict centers on the psychiatric nomenclature for homosexuality. In the first edition of the *Diagnostic and Statistical Manual* (the bible of psychiatric nomenclature) homosexuality was listed as a mental disorder. Books written predominantly by psychoanalysts were circulated widely among psychiatrists, providing guidelines for treating homosexuals with the explicit goal of changing their sexual orientation.[68] But the board of trustees of the APA removed homosexuality from the second edition of the *Diagnostic and Statistical Manual* in 1973, stating a lack of evidence showing that homosexuality meets criteria for a mental disorder. The third edition of the manual (DSM-III, 1980) included a diagnosis of ego-dystonic homosexuality, allowing a mental illness to be diagnosed if a person expressed a homosexual orientation yet was suffering significant internal conflict because of it. In 1984 ego-dystonic homosexuality was removed from DSM-III on the basis of lack of evidence that this condition is a mental disorder. In 1994 the APA took a further step, stating that it does not endorse any psychiatric treatment based either on a psychiatrist's assumption that homosexuality is a mental disorder or on a psychiatrist's intent to change a person's sexual orientation, even when the patient desires such treatment.[69] This position is difficult for evangelical psychiatrists, and they have challenged APA representatives to change the statement.[70]

Evangelical Christians challenge homosexual behavior not on the basis that it is a disease but based on the conviction that it is morally wrong. Evangelical Christian psychiatrists fear the recent actions of the American Psychiatric Association because of the potential impact on their practices. If persons with a homosexual orientation seek help from Christian psychiatrists to control their homosexual behavior because they (the patients) believe it to be morally wrong, are the psychiatrists prohibited from using their professional skills to assist these persons in seeking their treatment goals? In like manner, if a woman seeks advice from an evangelical psychiatrist regarding psychological consequences of abortion, must the psychiatrist state that there are no adverse psychological consequences? The positions taken in this debate are by their nature political (regardless of who is right or wrong), and a political battle does not encourage meaningful conversation.

Once these issues enter the political arena, the anxieties, concerns and values of the individual patient and psychiatrist often get lost in the wars of two opposing political groups. I believe it is possible for therapists to engage in a meaningful dialogue about an issue such as homosexuality and homosexual behavior with patients/counselees as long as the therapists are clear about taking a particular stand. For example, I believe I have engaged in beneficial conversation with avowed homosexuals who know from the outset my belief that homosexual behavior is wrong. These conversations did not lapse into doctrinal debates, yet they did not require me to compromise my beliefs either. The persons with whom I worked sought me out *because* they know I believe differently from them. The willingness to engage in dialogue with someone with a different belief was the beginning of the therapeutic relationship. In addition, I believe my patients and I have both learned from these therapeutic sessions.

A complicating factor is whether an insurance company should pay for therapy grounded in evangelical Christian values. As virtually all psychiatric therapy now is "subsidized" through insurance companies and federal insurance plans, such as Medicare and Medicaid, the issue of diagnosis involves government and politics. A political debate is not a philosophical or theological debate. Political confrontations may produce winners and losers but often do not significantly inform either side. Neither psychiatry nor evangelical Christianity can resolve these issues by political means to the satisfaction of the other. The law and politics have too often collaborated with American society in trivializing religious values. Stephen Carter, a Christian professor of law at Yale, says, "In our sensible zeal to keep religion from dominating our politics, we have created a political and legal culture that presses the religiously faithful to be other than themselves, to act publicly, and sometimes privately as well, as though their faith does not matter to them."[71]

The APA, in its policy pronouncements, is responding to the political and legal culture, not our actual knowledge regarding the sensitive issues of abortion and homosexuality. Scientific evidence that truly informs psychiatry to take a strong stand on either side of these issues is not currently available and, I suspect, will never be available. Therefore a "scientific" discussion of such issues is perhaps impossible. A meaningful conversation must take root in mutual respect: psychiatrists need to respect Christian values, and evangelicals need to understand and respect the culture of psychiatry and the values implicit in it.

Evangelical Christian counselors are suspect when they suggest that personal conflicts and emotional suffering can be solved by profamily votes at the ballot box. What happens to the individual in the process? A story from early Christian writings illustrates Jesus' recognition of the futility of legal and ethical pronouncements for solving the emotional and spiritual problems of individuals. Persons attempting to trap Jesus in a political debate brought to him a woman who had been caught sleeping with a man who was not her husband. They said, "Teacher, this woman was caught in the act of adultery. In the Law Moses commanded us to stone such women. Now what do you say?"

If Jesus said they should obey the law of Moses and stone the woman, he would be challenging Roman law. He himself had stated that his followers should submit themselves to Roman law. But if, on the other hand, he indicated that the law of Moses no longer applied, he would be contradicting another of his pronouncements, that he had come to fulfill the law of Moses rather than abolish it.

Jesus instead cut to the real problem. The woman was being treated as an object of theological/political debate rather than as a person. Turning to those challenging him, he said, "If anyone of you is without sin, let him be the first to throw a stone at her. " His challengers walked away, and Jesus turned to the woman, saying that since no one remained to condemn her, he did not condemn her either. Nevertheless, he encouraged her to take a good look at her life and lead a more moral life (Jn 8:2-11).

Jesus did not lose his mind in the heat of the crisis. He did not permit the political debate between the Romans and the Jews to distract him from his purpose of reaching out to those suffering spiritually and emotionally. The early church similarly deemphasized politics and emphasized a healing relationship with persons who were suffering.

Christian counselors today have, in my opinion, lost this focus. They would rather argue a clear and unambiguous doctrine in the public arena than deal with the more ambiguous and complex emotional problems experienced by individual Christians relating to one another and to the counselor. They have revolted against the complexities of the modern age with cut-and-dried moral pronouncements and simple prescriptions for complicated problems.

As I reflect on my conversations with the members of my faith community, I find myself longing to speak with my grandparents, the conservative Christians who read and wrote those marginal notes in the books I inherited. I realize I have projected my own interests and desires on my grandparents, whom I never actually knew. I also realize that I am perhaps being unfair to my Christian friends because my interests and concerns are not the same as theirs. I see the worst problems, the difficult cases, and so may have a different perspective. I also have been fortunate to have a family that has remained intact, not plagued by problems such as drug abuse and violence. I have been fortunate to receive an income that has been more than adequate for the needs of my family. We, as a family, have experienced emotional pain, yet we have worked through it. In other words, I have been blessed with the emotional freedom to confront these problems. If my children were daily being challenged or threatened as they attend school, if I saw one of my children falling apart emotionally and felt powerless to correct the problem, perhaps I would be attracted to the simplistic solutions I read in many books produced by the Christian counseling industry. Perhaps I would be attracted to the promises of the Christian political right. The thoughtful, intelligent approach I believe was taken by my grandparents was perhaps an illusion, or perhaps my grandparents were highly unusual.

Even so, something is missing from the approach taken by the Christian community in its ministry to the emotional pain experienced by its members. Of this I am convinced. I believe a good portion of what is missing is a commitment to probe to the depth of real-life problems, wherever that leads us. We cannot hide from the complex realities that underlie severe emotional pain.

Thoughtful Christian service is hard work, work in the trenches of difficult helping relationships. The benefits of this work come slowly. Understanding of persons with emotional pain comes slowly. Finding ways to help others out of their pain takes even more effort and will not always endear us to our Christian companions.

Once a community becomes complacent in its approach to tough problems, it does not easily change. I believe many evangelical Christians, especially Christian counselors, have taken an easy, mindless path. Critical thinking about emotional suffering in the Christian community is discouraged. Christianity has lost its mind when it comes to helping persons with severe emotional problems.

5

Filling the Vacuum

I *believe both psychiatrists and* Christians want to talk. In fact, I have been testing the possibilities, and I am getting a response. The response, however, is vague. I feel more as if I am being pulled into a vacuum than attracted to a specific topic of conversation. Psychiatrists and Christians don't know where to begin a conversation to which both are attracted.

Some, however, are beginning to fill that vacuum, to speak from the vacuum. Though these persons are to some extent on the fringe of psychiatry and/or Christianity, they are speaking and writing from the center of something. Is this something central to understanding the severe emotional pain felt by the searching schizophrenic Barbara or the confused and depressed Jason (see chapter one)? I believe the answer is yes. Have these persons completed the task and answered the questions that prompted me to write this book? No. I believe they have only begun to fill the vacuum. Many more psychiatrists and Christians must join the conversation if the vacuum is to be filled. Yet we can learn from those at the fringe who have recognized the vacuum and worked to fill it.

In this chapter I review some movements that, in my opinion, attempt to fill the vacuum in our society to which persons with emotional problems and the people who care for them gravitate. These movements, in large part, did not originate as a result of the lack of conversation between psychiatry and Christianity but as a reaction to general trends in our society. These diverse movements have not emerged predominantly to heal the psychiatrically ill. Nevertheless, each has influenced persons with emotional problems and the people who care for them. These movements include the reemergence of patient-centered care among nonpsychiatric physicians, the New Age and renewed emphasis on the spiritual, "soul doctors," self-help groups, and narrative theology.

What do they have in common? I believe they have soul and mind. By "soul" I mean that they focus on relationships with others and/or the transcendent. They have "mind" in the sense that they provide a fresh (though not always tight) argument that something is missing in our understanding of and care for emotional suffering. In this brief review I am not able to describe all movements that address the vacuum. The writers I mention are not necessarily the best, yet they are writers who have caught my attention and the attention of others and have made us think.

Patient-Centered Care Among Nonpsychiatric Physicians

There is a movement afoot in medicine to focus again on the patient. The new technologies of medicine, the pressure to be more time-efficient and the loss of the once-cherished doctor-patient relationship have all contributed to a desire among physicians to reestablish patient-centered care. The disappearance of the special relationship between the family doctor and persons in his or her community has been as disturbing to physicians as to the patients they treat. Popular writers such as Norman Cousins and Reynolds Price have pointed out the insensitivity of some modern doctors. Price, in *A Whole New Life: An Illness and a Healing,* emphasizes the lack of concern he felt from a radiation therapist who treated him for a cancer of his spinal column: "The most grueling treatment . . . would be presided over by a radiation oncologist who gave the unbroken impression, over five weeks, of being nothing so much as a nuclear physicist whose experimental subjects were, sadly for them, human beings."[1]

That professionals from any discipline can discharge the responsibilities of their profession solely on the basis of precise science has been challenged by the social scientist Donald Schon.[2] He suggests that the best professionals know more than they can put into words; they rely less on algorithms or formulas learned during their professional training than on an intuitive "improvisation" learned during their practice. Schon labels this approach to practice "reflection-in-action." One characteristic of the practice of a professional is that the professional approaches each problem as a unique case, a unique relationship. Though the doctor calls upon prior relevant experiences, the effective practitioner recognizes the peculiarities of the situation at hand. Standard solutions are secondary to specific solutions that are based on individuals rather than the aggregated experimental subjects suggested by Price; they are "case based." Perhaps cased-based means "Let me, the patient, tell you as my physician about myself as well as my illness. You need to know my soul to care for my illness."

Case-based or patient-centered care requires doctors to understand illness through the eyes of the patient. Margaret Gerteis and her colleagues in health care research, in *Through the Patient's Eyes,* have suggested a conceptual framework for patient-centered medical practice which emphasizes respect for a patient's values, preferences and expressed needs; physical comfort of the patient; emotional support and the alleviation of fear and anxiety; the involvement of family and friends; and the perspective of working with patients and families through time.[3] Questions the physician should ask in order to promote patient-centered therapy include "What impact does the illness or treatment have on the patient's quality of life or subjective sense of well-being?" "How is the illness and treatment mediated by life-style, cultural values, and religious beliefs?" "Are patients treated with dignity, respect, and sensitivity to their cultural values?"[4] Gerteis and her colleagues therefore acknowledge the spiritual, yet the spiritual is not central.

Perhaps the physician who has emphasized patient-centered therapy most vocally is Eric Cassel. In *The Nature of Suffering and the Goals of Medicine,* Cassel emphasizes the centrality of the patient for understanding suffering. "The test of a system of medicine should be its adequacy in the face of suffering. . . . Bodies do not suffer, persons suffer. . . . Modern medicine is too devoted to its science and technology and has lost touch with the personal side of sickness."[5] Cardiologists, surgeons and radiologists, as well as primary care physicians, have expressed new interest in improving the doctor-patient relationship and in understanding patients' suffering.

One important aspect of patient-centered therapy is permitting the patient to tell his or her own story (which I return to later in discussing narrative theology). Psychiatrist/anthropologist Arthur Kleinman, in *Illness Narratives: Suffering, Healing and the Human Condition,* argues that interpreting the illness experience is an art tragically neglected by modern medical training and suggests that narrative is a key to bridging the gap between the patient and the practitioner.[6]

> The interpretation of narratives of illness experience is a core task in the work of doctoring. . . . Illness has meaning; and to understand how it obtains meaning is to understand something fundamental about illness, about care, and perhaps about life generally. Moreover, an interpretation of illness is something that patients, families, and practitioners need to undertake together.[7]

I find it encouraging yet disturbing as a psychiatrist to witness the reemergence of interest among my colleagues of other specialties in the doctor-patient relationship, patient-centered care and the emphasis on allowing the patient to tell her or his story. The psychiatrist has, in many medical schools, faded to the background among physicians who teach the medical student how to talk with and listen to the patient. The internist, the pediatrician and the family physician have moved to fill the vacuum. Patients suffering physical and emotional illness feel the need to be heard—a need well expressed by Price and William Styron (see chapter two). As a medical educator I have confidence that in the future physicians will respond better to their patients, despite the changes occurring in our health care system. Patients will demand patient-centered care, and doctors will rediscover that the joy of practicing medicine derives from the practice of patient-centered care. Even so, I fear psychiatrists may not be at the forefront of the reemergence of patient-centered care.

I also fear the church has not facilitated this movement. The Christian church has much to teach doctors about the meaning of illness to Christians, primarily because the church should be caring for the souls of its members. A pastor, an elder or priest is often the person to whom those suffering physical and emotional illness first turn. Unfortunately, the church today is likely to provide only static, formula-driven responses to its members or to express inability to understand the complexities of an illness and its healing. The church prefers to prescribe and refer rather than to listen. The Christian community, if it is to be effective, must develop skills to listen and share in the interpretation of illness narratives. The church must be as patient-centered as the physician.

I fear Christian counselors frequently avoid patient-centered care. They find it far more comfortable to take a detached, prescriptive approach to those experiencing emotional suffering, an approach that often manifests itself in listening too little and advising too much. Giving advice often does not require becoming involved emotionally.

The New Age Movement

In the midst of advancing technologies and an emphasis on the brain among psychiatrists, a movement of spiritual openness has emerged in American society. Even as some scientists/philosophers suggest "the mind is the brain,"[8] others are reacting dramatically to this monist-materialist view of the mind. This movement in search of spirituality ranges widely. The lead article in *Newsweek* on November 28, 1994, explored the renewed search for the sacred: "Maybe it's a critical mass of baby boomers in the contemplative afternoon of life, or anxiety over the millennium, or a general dissatisfaction with the materialism of the modern world. For these reasons and more, millions of Americans are embarking on a search for the sacred in their lives."[9] Though some have sought the spiritual by a return to traditional religion, many others have sought the spiritual outside the Judeo-Christian-Islamic tradition. "Spiritual" is perhaps an impossible concept to define in relation to this current trend. Few would deny, however, that the "search" is a quest for relationship, for understanding oneself in the context of a larger social and even cosmic context.

Nontraditional explorations of the spiritual and metaphysical have been loosely described as the New Age movement. Characteristics of this movement include a look to the East for inspiration; emphasis on meditation and self-control, or the spiritual over the physical; and advocacy of a different type of monism—the unity of life rather than distinctions between Creator and created.[10] New Age philosophy transcends history, is pluralistic and experiential, and is expressive rather than rule-oriented. Private life, especially private spiritual life, is the emphasis, as opposed to public responsibility or group joining. Yet this emphasis on private spiritual lives derives, in my opinion, from a sense of isolation. The New Age is thought to be a reaction to our depersonalized, technological society, which treats individuals as interchangeable parts. Therefore the New Age movement, in a somewhat perverted way, attempts to counteract the sense of isolation and depersonalization by encouraging the person to "get in touch with yourself" and to find unity and meaning through self-integration.

Though the New Age movement deemphasizes the historical, it may not be all that new for Americans. It is the descendant of Ralph Waldo Emerson's transcendentalism.[11] Emerson championed self-development and focused on the unique resources in each individual. Emerson took his views of self-reliance beyond the idea of pulling yourself up by your own bootstraps. In his view there is a correspondence between humankind and everything in the universe. He took an intuitive, experiential rather than rational approach to reality. Self-development includes spiritual development—a unique American form of spiritual development.

This drive for spiritual development via the self, however, falls short of its goal. A common thread among New Age enthusiasts is the pursuit of an elevated consciousness. This pursuit is exemplified in the writings and practices of the actress Shirley MacLaine. Christianity is viewed as being irrelevant to the New Age, because the god for the New Age must be immanent in both outward nature and consciousness. There is no intervening space for incarnation.[12] The immanent "god" of New Age practices, however, is far from isolating. For example, interests as far-ranging as reincarnation, Satanism and Buddhism imply relationship. If one peruses the New Age section at a bookstore, books on reincarnation, witchcraft,

Satanism, meditation and Zen Buddhist practices are included.

How is the New Age relevant to the conversation between psychiatry and Christianity? First, psychiatry has deemphasized the metaphysical in its pursuit of physical causes of serious emotional problems. The persons who experience these problems, however, perceive them to be, at least in part, the result of spiritual sickness or emptiness and are frustrated with materialistic approaches to their problems. (Jason, in chapter one, sought a spiritual explanation of his illness, though his search did not take him in the direction of the New Age.) They rebel against the belief that all mental phenomena can be explained by neurobiological mechanisms and that all experiences can be reduced to physiochemical phenomena. If they turn to traditional religion, especially turn-of-the-millennium evangelical Christianity, they are more likely to find mechanistic prescriptions for behavioral change than a conversation edifying the soul. So they seek nourishment for their hungry souls elsewhere.

The dissatisfaction of some psychiatric patients explains only a small portion of the impetus for the New Age Movement. American religion historically has been a religion of individuality that permits one to commune with God freely. "Accept Jesus into your heart" is a call to a private faith, not open to the scrutiny of others. It is a call to a faith that transcends authority, especially the authority of the church. It is a call that brings God close as a personal friend rather than rejecting him as a transcendent being. It is a religion that, at least as prescribed by some, requires little of its followers. In other words, there is an immanent theme in traditional American religion upon which the New Age movement has capitalized, albeit in a much modified form. The increasing diversity of American society undoubtedly contributes to the popularity of New Age thinking as well.

Those who seek something more fit no particular profile and therefore travel many and varied pathways to the new spirituality. The American religious establishment appears painfully restrictive to those seeking a "true religious experience," and this restriction has led them to seek alternative means to express their religious sentiments. Some evangelical churches have been increasingly associated with conservative, limiting politics and doctrine with little room for diversity. The traditions of mainline Protestant

Christianity appear sterile and archaic. Persons in mental anguish who feel a need for healing of soul often find themselves frustrated or constrained within established Christianity and therefore seek New Age approaches to spirituality where responsibilities are limited, doctrines are virtually non-existent and the individual is free to find soul in her or his own way. Every experience is a real one, whether it be a near-death experience or reincarnation.

Though the New Age Movement did not arise to fill the vacuum left by the absence of a conversation between psychiatry and Christianity, though it is perhaps a natural evolution of American culture and religion, it does fill a void for many who suffer emotionally and seek care of the soul. Those attracted to the New Age therefore move away from both traditional psychiatry and Christianity.

The New Age provides an opportunity for conversation between psychiatry and Christianity, yet both must enter new territory and grapple with a language that is unfamiliar. For example, the New Age commonly uses the language of the "spiritual." Psychiatrists are especially uncomfortable when speaking of the spiritual, given their recent push toward an objective science of the mind/brain based in observable phenomena—that is, the material. Many evangelical Christians are equally uncomfortable discussing the spiritual with those involved in New Age, especially when "spiritual" implies concepts such as reincarnation and Satanism.

Still, many persons experiencing emotional suffering use New Age language to express their anguish and their hopes. Psychiatrists and evangelical Christians could engage in a useful dialogue focused on meaningful communication with persons not firmly grounded in established scientific or religious constructs of their pain.

The Soul Doctors
A number of therapists have virtually severed their identity with their professional disciplines, whether that discipline be psychiatry, clinical psychology or pastoral counseling, and have identified themselves as doctors of soul. Perhaps the best known of these therapists of recent years are Thomas Moore and M. Scott Peck. In *Care of the Soul*[13] (which reached

number one on the *New York Times* bestseller list) Moore provides a guide
for cultivating "depth and sacredness in everyday life." He encourages
persons to let up on themselves, that is, to lower their expectations. They
have placed excessive pressure on themselves to lose weight, to become
more emotionally independent, to release themselves from long-term anger
at parents and to leave a less-than-perfect job or marriage. Opportunities
can be found in suffering, problems will never cease, and therefore Moore
encourages persons to enjoy life rather than work so hard to improve
themselves. He encourages persons to be comfortable with themselves in
relationship to others and to nourish and be nourished by others.

Moore comes from an eclectic background, having studied for the
priesthood and completed a bachelor's degree in theology, philosophy and
musicology. He gained expertise in classical literature and the Italian
Renaissance as well as knowledge of Eastern religions. He is a "practicing
Zen-influenced Jungian," with the goal of inserting the spiritual into psychology.

When Moore describes soul, he takes care not to ally himself with a
specific philosophical or religious system, but he believes spiritual wisdom
can be derived from many cultures. Rather than attempting the difficult task
of defining soul, he encourages the person suffering emotional problems to
feel soul in order to know it. As with beauty and pleasure, an individual
recognizes the soul when she or he encounters it.

Moore believes that the popularity of his book and his approach derive
from a general dissatisfaction in society with the narcissism of the 1980s
and the emphasis on improving economic well-being. Persons of the 1990s
realize that satisfaction must go deeper, and self-reflection has come much
more into vogue. Moore suggests that certain emotional problems can be
spiritual gifts: "In a society that is defended against the tragic sense of life,
depression will appear as an enemy, an unredeemable malady; yet in such
a society, devoted to light, depression, in compensation, will be unusually
strong."[14]

Moore specifically emphasizes the need of the soul for what he calls
"vernacular life," a relationship to a local place and culture. "It [the soul]
has a preference for details and particulars, intimacy and involvement,

attachment and rootedness."[15] He encourages persons who wish to care for their souls to engage in religious rituals that enable them to root themselves in spiritual communities and retreat from the modern world. Moore thus has recognized a void among those suffering emotionally and prescribes many solutions that traditionally were rooted in the Christian church and pastoral care. Today, however, he stands apart from both the church and mainstream psychotherapy.

Psychiatrist M. Scott Peck is another doctor of soul. His 1978 book *The Road Less Traveled: A New Psychology of Love, Traditional Values and Spiritual Growth* has been an inspiration for thousands of persons seeking relief from emotional suffering.[16] Peck, though trained as a psychiatrist, has not been firmly rooted in either psychiatry or mainline Christianity (even though he embraced Christianity soon after publishing *The Road Less Traveled*). Even so, he has gathered a following among mainline and evangelical Christians. Like Moore, he draws on many sources, including Eastern religions, in developing his approach to psychotherapy.

In his writing Peck makes two assumptions. First, there is no distinction between the mind and the spirit, and therefore no distinction between the process of achieving spiritual growth and that of achieving mental growth. Second, the process of psychotherapy, and therefore mental and spiritual growth, is a complex, arduous and lifelong task. Psychotherapy, if it is to provide substantial assistance to the process of mental and spiritual growth, is not a quick or simple procedure. "I do not believe there are any single easy answers. I believe that brief forms of psychotherapy may be helpful and are not to be decried, but the help they provide is inevitably superficial."[17]

Peck therefore emphasizes the importance of spending adequate time with the person suffering emotional problems and permitting the story of the individual to unfold over time. In this emphasis Peck reflects a central characteristic of psychoanalysis: the importance of the patient's story, told in confidence built over time with the therapist. Psychiatry has wandered far from this emphasis. The cost of therapy in a time of cost containment undoubtedly has contributed to the change in orientation of traditional psychiatry, but as noted throughout this book, there have been other factors within and without that have led psychiatrists away from long-term, in-depth relationships with their patients. Peck prescribes time together to fill this void left by the illusion of "quick solutions."

Peck also emphasizes the importance of religion but, like Moore, takes a eclectic approach to it. "Among the members of the human race there exists an extraordinary variability in the breadth and sophistication of our understanding of what life is about. This understanding is our religion. Since everyone has some understanding—some world view, no matter how limited, primitive or inaccurate—everyone has a religion."[18] Peck goes on to criticize modern psychiatrists: "In supervising other psychotherapists, I rather routinely find that they pay too little, if any, attention to the ways in which their patients view the world. . . . So I say to those I supervise: 'Find out your patients' religions even if they say they don't have any.' "[19]

Like Moore, Peck views emotional suffering, especially depression, as an opportunity for growth. "The act of deciding to seek psychiatric attention in itself represents giving up of the self-image 'I'm OK.' . . . The feeling associated with giving up something loved—or at least something that is a part of ourselves and familiar—is depression."[20] For Peck, depression is a healthy phenomenon and becomes unhealthy only when it is prolonged. Depression enables persons to honestly reflect on themselves in the context of their relationships with others and their religious sentiments.

Other doctors of soul have maintained their identity within mainstream psychiatry or psychology, yet have broken traditional paradigms within the ranks. The psychiatrist Irving Yalom, in his book *Existential Psychotherapy*, attempted to take psychiatry in a direction quite opposed to trends of the time.[21] Yalom, unlike Moore and Peck, was a respected academic psychiatrist, a member of the faculty at Stanford University School of Medicine. He is one of the country's leading experts in group psychotherapy. His exposition of existential therapy represents more an evolution from traditional Freudian psychotherapy than a revolution. Nevertheless, the constructs Yalom emphasizes were put forward to fill a void he perceived in the psychotherapy practiced during the late 1970s, even the psychotherapies based in Freudian psychoanalysis. He describes his expanded approach as "a framework for many of the extras of therapy" and recognizes that existential psychotherapy defies definition but is an approach to therapy that emphasizes concerns rooted in the individual's existence.[22]

The concept of existential psychotherapy did not originate with Yalom. Existential therapists, or at least therapists expressing an existential orientation, such as Rollo May, Carl Rogers, Fritz Perls and Abraham Maslow, were prevalent and popular during the 1950s and 1960s. The roots of existential therapy reach back to a time almost parallel to the emergence of psychoanalysis.

Ludwig Binswanger, an early psychoanalyst strongly influenced by the German philosopher Martin Heidegger, made a probing criticism of psychoanalysis during the 1940s.[23] Though Binswanger remained loyal to Freud, he believed Freud fell short in considering the existential and self-realization as expressions of humankind's capacity for Being. He especially criticized the reductive method of psychoanalysis with its roots in the natural sciences and encouraged analysts to move from phenomenology to "existential ontology." Rather than attributing psychopathology to disturbances of disposition or constitution, Binswanger emphasized disturbances of specific "world design" or continuity. "The particular world design, in accordance with which each human being enters life, is comparable to the philosophical categories, i.e., to a priori structures."[24] The therapist therefore should not attempt to explain the emotional suffering of the patient in accordance with the doctrines of a specific school of psychiatry but should understand that suffering as a modification of the total structure of "being-in-the-world." Therapy, likewise, is grounded in the relationship of the patient and therapist within that "being-in-the-world."

Yalom expands on this theme, which had run parallel to traditional psychoanalysis (and therefore traditional psychiatry). During the 1940s and 1950s a dialogue was maintained between transitional psychoanalysis and existential analysis. This dialogue virtually disappeared after the mid-twentieth century. Yalom addresses four existential issues: death, freedom, isolation and meaninglessness. He suggests that existential isolation refers to "an unbridgeable gulf between one's self and any other being . . . a separation between the individual and the world."[25] In his therapeutic approach to existential isolation, Yalom emphasizes the importance of the patient-doctor relationship. "It's the relationship that heals."[26] Yalom breaks tradition with the psychoanalyst, however, by asserting the need to make the doctor-patient relationship a "real" relationship. Specifically, he encourages doctors to open themselves to their patients rather than keep their distance in order to analyze the response of the patient or feelings the patient transfers to therapy from previous experiences.

A singular focus on transference impedes therapy because it precludes an authentic therapist-patient relationship. First, it negates the reality of the relationship by considering the relationship solely as a key to understanding a more important relationship. Secondly, it provides the therapist with a rationale for personal concealment.[27]

Yalom goes further by emphasizing love as a facilitator of growth. "One of the outstanding characteristics of 'psychotherapeutic eros' is the care for the other's becoming. . . . What is important, then, is that therapist self-disclosure be in the service of the growth of the patient."[28]

Yalom calls for therapists to be genuine and open and to consider every aspect of the patient's being. Though he does not emphasize religion, as do Moore and Peck, he clearly recognizes the importance of religion in helping the individual to define meaning, specifically the purpose of one's life. Yalom does not recommend that the therapist attack meaninglessness head-on with discussions of religious doctrines or cosmic views of the universe. He suggests that meaning derives from engagement, from relationship.

Meaning, like pleasure, must be pursued obliquely. A sense of meaningfulness is a by-product of engagement. . . . Engagement is the therapeutic answer to meaninglessness regardless of the latter's source. . . . To find a home, to care about other individuals, about ideas or projects, to search, to create, to build—these, and all other forms of engagement, are twice rewarding: they're intrinsically enriching, and they alleviate the dysphoria that stems from being bombarded with the unassembled data of existence.[29]

Like Moore and Peck, Yalom seeks guidance and depth from the wisdom of religions, literature and philosophy of the world. At the conclusion of his book he distinguishes existential therapy from usual therapies because it is humanistically based and, alone among therapeutic paradigms, is entirely concordant with the intensively personal nature of the therapeutic enterprise. Moreover, the existential paradigm has a broad sweep: it gathers and harvests the insights of many philosophers, artists, and therapists about the painful and redemptive confrontation with ultimate concerns.[30]

From the perspective of one thoroughly trained in traditional psychiatric therapies and firmly rooted within the psychiatric establishment, this book is exceptional both for its content and for its timing. *Existential Psychotherapy* never became a bestseller among psychiatrists but has gained an audience in the nonpsychiatric community. Unlike Viktor Frankl (see chapter four), who addressed similar issues, Yalom has not gained a wide following among Christian counselors. Frankl resonated with Christians because he searched for meaning outside the mundane, a meaning from relationship. Yalom does speak, however, to issues that are of great concern to persons who feel a vacuum in current approaches to the treatment of emotional suffering.

Robert Coles is a psychiatrist/anthropologist who received a Pulitzer Prize for his study of children in the South during the 1960s. Though Coles has always been willing to explore at the fringe of mainstream psychiatry, in recent years he has focused much more on the spiritual. He struggled with the tension between psychoanalysis and religion through his study of children. In the introduction to his book *The Spiritual Life of Children,* Coles writes, "Before I could let children begin to teach me a few lessons, I had to look inward and examine my own assumptions about religion as a psychological phenomenon and as a social and historical force."[31] Unlike Yalom, Coles has not developed a therapy for soul. Yet his willingness to reveal his own inner struggles as he carries on the conversation between psychiatry and religion is a model for psychiatrists and Christian therapists. Coles, however, has not received as much attention recently as in the past within mainstream psychiatry, and his psychospiritual explorations deviate dramatically from neuropsychiatry.

Yet another individual whose work has addressed the vacuum is Allen Bergin, a psychologist at Brigham Young University. In 1980 Bergin wrote a seminal article for the *Journal of Consulting in Clinical Psychology* entitled "Psychotherapy and Religious Values."[32] What renders Bergin unique is that he published a challenging article, a debate really, in a respected psychological journal regarding the interaction of psychology and religion. He argued that religion should be considered more empirically and systematically in personality theories and therapeutic interventions. In other words, the psychotherapeutic treatment of persons cannot be divorced from their cultural context. Bergin was immediately challenged by a well-known psychologist, Albert Ellis. "Religiosity is in many respects equivalent to irrational thinking in an emotional disturbance. . . . The elegant therapeutic solution to emotional problems is to be quite unreligious. . . . The less religious they are, the more emotionally healthy they will be."[33]

This type of heated exchange in a respected psychological journal is unusual today. Bergin stoked the embers of a dying fire and has continued to argue his position in traditional psychological journals.[34] He proposes that values and ideology influence theoretical axioms; conceptions of personality and psychopathology have subjective as well as empirical bases. Mental health literature and education are limited by their minimal appreciation for the religious subcultures of our society, and religious factors either are excluded from management or are included in such a way as to prejudice the results.[35]

As described in chapter three, Bergin's argument for a review of the empirical literature that is more fair to religion is joined by other social scientists. Even the U.S. government is listening. The National Institute on Aging held a conference in March 1995 to discuss the relationship of religion and health among the elderly and to stimulate additional empirical research.

Bergin's call for more honest empirical research is not unique. For example, the Association for Spiritual, Ethical and Religious Values publishes a peer-reviewed journal, *Counseling and Values*. Typical titles of articles include "Therapist Spiritual and Religious Values In Psychotherapy," "Integrating Religious Experiences in Counseling," "Self-Transcendence: Integrating Ends and Means in Valued Counseling" and "Religious Counseling: To Be Used, Not Feared." The journal publishes articles on issues of importance to counselors who recognize the spiritual sterility of modern psychotherapy. The active participants in this association and contributors to the publication have not strongly identified themselves with any religious group (though they are predominantly Protestant Christians) and have, to some extent, left the mainstream of psychology. What sets them apart from the Christian counseling industry described in chapter four is the attempt to integrate psychology and religion as scholars.

This group has not attempted to write for the lay public and does not readily adopt psychological and psychiatric theories that happen to be in vogue, but questions these theories and therapies. Bergin is a model for this group of thoughtful practitioners; generally every article in the journal includes at least one reference to Bergin. Other scholars referred to frequently by contributors to the journal are Robert Bellah and his colleagues, sociologists who challenged the individualism and isolation of contemporary American society in *Habits of the Heart.* The journal is also conspicuous for the absence of references to articles by the best-known participants in the Christian counseling industry, such James Dobson, Frank Minirth, Paul Meier, Tim LaHaye and David Seamands. The association appears to meet a need for academic discussion of the relationship between psychology and the values of faith communities. Strongly influenced by psychologists, it has emphasized psychotherapy with little discussion of value issues regarding biological therapies. Rarely, if ever, do psychiatrists publish in this journal. The emergence of this association helps fill a void felt by many academically oriented psychologists and Christian theologians/counselors.

The construct of "spirit" may serve as a bridge psychiatrists and evangelical Christians can employ to connect with persons involved in the New Age. In the same manner, the construct of "soul," as employed by writers such as Thomas Moore, is a bridge to many persons who are seeking something to heal their emotional suffering beyond the scientific and beyond traditional religion. There is considerable overlap between New Age concepts of spirit and the current interest in soul, and no clear line of demarcation can be employed. Yet soul, or the absence of soul, provides an excellent point of contact as psychiatrists and evangelical Christians seek to reach the emotionally suffering. Persons suffering express, in many and varied ways (as illustrated above), that traditional psychiatry and evangelical Christianity just do not reach the "heart and soul" of their suffering.

Self-Help Groups

Self-help groups have become ubiquitous in Western society. The impetus for developing these groups and their value to society far exceeds the vacuum produced by a lack of conversation between psychiatry and Christianity. Nevertheless, certain characteristics of self-help groups highlight the absence of this conversation. Two self-help movements are illustrative, though many others could be described.

Alcoholics Anonymous (AA) was established in 1935 and is today perhaps the most useful organization in the United States to assist persons suffering from alcohol abuse and dependence. AA operates much like a religious community, complete with doctrine. The twelve steps proposed as necessary to overcome alcoholism reflect a creed that shapes AA as much as any creed shapes a religious group and have strong religious overtones. These steps include the following:

☐ We admit we are powerless over alcohol—that our lives have become unmanageable.

☐ We have come to believe that a Power greater than ourselves can restore us to sanity.

☐ We have made a decision to turn our will and our lives over to the care of God as we understand him.

☐ We seek through prayer and meditation to improve our conscientious contact with God as we understand him, praying only for the knowledge of his will for us and the power to carry that out.

These steps are virtually identical to the cognitive-behavioral approach used by the Christian counseling industry to treat alcohol and drug abuse. In fact, the Christian counseling industry has appropriated this twelve-step approach as a Christian treatment.

Nevertheless, Alcoholics Anonymous accomplishes something that most religious groups and Christian counselors have great difficulty in accomplishing; it provides a strong, supportive community that has great influence over the individual. In most U.S. towns and cities of any size Alcoholics

Anonymous meetings are available seven days a week, and a newly absti-
nent alcoholic is encouraged to attend ninety meetings in ninety days. The
key to the success of Alcoholics Anonymous is unambivalently available
support to the alcoholic from persons who have similar problems. Even after
months and years of abstinence, participants will attend two or three AA
meetings a week and take it upon themselves to care for and serve persons
who newly join AA or who have relapsed into alcohol abuse. A new member
has available a telephone number of an experienced AA member twenty-
four hours a day, seven days a week, and the group is known for its
willingness to rush to the aid of a person who is struggling to refrain from
taking a drink.

A second group filling the void is the Samaritans. This group also has
been in existence for over forty years, primarily in the United Kingdom.
They typically respond to 2.5 million contacts each year and have two
hundred branches with 23,500 volunteers.[36] The Samaritans make themselves available by telephone twenty-four hours a day, by personal visits
during the daytime and evening, and also by letter. The seven principles and
practices of the Samaritans state, for example, that help is to be confidential,
nonjudgmental and nonadvisory; no spiritual-political-philosophic opinion
is to be pushed; and the individual and his or her feelings are to be fully
accepted. The group is available to assist persons struggling with a variety
of problems ranging from financial difficulties to contemplation of suicide.
The Samaritans differ from Alcoholics Anonymous in that their volunteers
do not necessarily have the problems experienced by those whom they
serve. The bonding of the Samaritans to persons in trouble is bonding the
troubled person to the group, not to any individual within the group (as
bonding individual to individual is key to the success of Alcoholics Anonymous). The Samaritans share a key characteristic with Alcoholics Anonymous: "we're always there."

In the best of all possible worlds, the church should serve this role. Its
troubled members should be as willing and as comfortable calling on the
resources of the church as they are calling on AA or the Samaritans. The
church's inability to provide such supportive services, however, partly led
to the emergence of these volunteer self-help groups. Many persons are

active in their churches while at the same time working with groups such as AA and Samaritans. The supportive services provided by AA and the Samaritans have rarely been well integrated into churches, though many churches have attempted to develop alcohol and drug abuse support groups and "hotlines" for the general public. Psychiatrists are most aware of the value of groups such as AA and therefore understand them, accept them and maintain a conversation with them. The conversation between psychiatry and Christianity would be strengthened if the church could be counted on to be there. The church is not always there, and psychiatrists know this well.

Narrative Theology

In recent years a lively debate has emerged among theologians[37] surrounding the appeal some have made to the importance of narrative and story. Stories have been used since antiquity as a means to guide Christians in ethics and theology. One reason is that story overcomes a barrier perceived by many: absolute principles, prescriptions and rules cannot serve as guides in and of themselves to Christian moral growth and development. Stanley Hauerwas, a proponent of narrative theology, states his case as follows: "What we need is not a principle or end but a narrative that charts a way for us to live coherently amid the diversity and conflicts that circumscribe and shape our moral existence."[38]

Like other movements described in this chapter, narrative theology did not emerge because of the lack of dialogue between psychiatry and Christianity. Rather, narrative theology addresses issues at the core of specialized debates within theology and ethics today. It does, however, reflect the vacuum between Christianity and psychiatry. Specifically, narrative theology suggests that suffering persons have lost their ability to understand and receive comfort by telling their story within a larger context. In other words, a person's story brings meaning to otherwise meaningless suffering.

Narrative theology has it roots earlier in the twentieth century, or at least it was "rediscovered" at this time. Richard Niebuhr (see chapter two) emphasized the importance of narrative and was one of the persons who brought it to the forefront in twentieth-century Christian theological discourse. In *The Meaning of Revelation* Niebuhr suggests that since ancient times story has been a key means by which Christians have interpreted meaning.

What prompted Christians in the past to confess their faith by telling the story of their life was more than a need for vivid illustration or for analogical reasoning. This story was not a parable which could be replaced by another; it was irreplaceable and untranslatable. An internal compulsion rather than free choice led them to speak of what they knew by telling them about Jesus Christ and their relation to God through him.[39] In other words, a person's story is the narrative of that person's relationship with his or her faith community through time, a relationship not only with community members but also with the larger story that shapes the community.

Discussions in narrative theology relate not only to the life history of the individual Christian but also to the historical narrative of the Christian community, the church. It is the interaction of the two, the individual story within the context of the larger story, that forms the heart of narrative theology. I suggest in chapter six that narrative is as important to finding meaning in emotional suffering as it is, according to its proponents, to finding meaning in Christian moral development. Niebuhr, for example, suggests that the individual Christian learns about his or her moral self within the context of feedback from the Christian community. Can the same be said for the emotional self?

Hauerwas, following this logic, believes that the development of the Christian life must occur within the community encouraged by a transformation of the self through direction from a master.[40] The Christian life therefore is best understood as a narrative, brought forth with the help of another who provides the skill to let persons claim their actions as their own. Our intentional actions are woven into the depiction of personal identity and character and become the language by which we describe our character and our behavior.[41]

Story, likewise, has been an integral part of twentieth-century psychiatry. Though the emphasis has been primarily on the life story of the individual, social psychiatrists at midcentury, such as Alexander Leighton, attempted to couple the story of the individual with the story of the community (see chapter six). These psychiatrists conceived emotional suffering in the context of community. The trajectory of a person's life history could not be abstracted from the life story of the community. For example, if an integrated community such as a cohesive fishing community in Nova Scotia evolved into an urban industrial center over the lifetime of a community resident, the changes in the community could not but affect the emotional well-being of that resident. In other words, social psychiatrists did not ignore the individual life stories on which psychoanalysts focused, but expanded the horizons of these stories to include the community as well.

Yet modern psychiatry has largely abandoned the story of the individual and almost exclusively abandoned the narrative of the community in which the individual resides. Time pressure has limited the telling of the stories by individuals. Perhaps the optimism of the 1960s, the era of the social psychiatrists, has given way to a resigned belief that societal ills cannot be changed and may only worsen. Therefore social concerns, let alone social activism, should be avoided.

Psychiatrists could benefit from a dialogue regarding social concern with evangelical Christians, who continue to believe the story of the community is important and can be modified by social action. Evangelical Christians could benefit from the dialogue through a healthy dose of realism.

The Need for Conversation

Throughout this book I have suggested that historical forces that have shaped psychiatry and Christianity (especially evangelical Christianity) have contributed to the absence of conversation between psychiatry and Christianity, the narrative of the dialogue. These forces include the emphasis on self to the exclusion of community, which has rendered the church less relevant as a source for healing emotional suffering to both the psychiatrist and the Christian counselor. Barbara (see chapter one) and her mother, from my perspective, experienced healing from the Christian community far more than from my assistance. Similarly, an emphasis on immediate gratification has undermined the patience necessary to "work through" one's story and one's suffering and has contributed to Christians' easy acceptance of individually prescribed self-help solutions for the relief of emotional suffering.

Psychiatrists and Christians to some extent have lost their intellectual curiosity regarding the questions psychiatry and religion naturally pose to one another, such as the role of relationship in healing the emotions. Psychiatrists don't read the religious classics that describe us in our narrative history. Christian counselors do not explore the philosophical underpinnings of modern neuropsychiatry and its tendency to isolate persons. Broad-based pastoral counseling and psychiatric theories at midcentury have given way to a specialization with blinders. Psychiatrists have become technicians and Christian counselors have become technocrats through the prescription of simplified formulas for living. The lack of conversation between psychiatrists and Christians can therefore be understood within the context of the history of relations between psychiatry and Christian theology/counseling. Is something missing, or are the trends we witness inevitable and therefore not to be challenged? I believe the above trends suggest something is missing.

Joseph English, past president of the American Psychiatric Association, apparently feels the same concern. A devout Catholic, English has challenged psychiatry to search for its own values again by returning to religious origins.

> Can our professional values be maintained without a conscious recognition of their origins in the Judeo-Christian tradition as well as the other great religions? Doesn't this suggest at least one reason why psychiatry and religion should be in a continuing and important dialogue? And despite our differences, is there not even the possibility of an alliance between psychiatry and religion related to values and objectives we share?[42]

English, like many of us in psychiatry, is searching for something more in the dialogue between psychiatry and Christianity than mere accommodation. Yet how can this something more be found? In the next chapter I suggest an approach to beginning a serious conversation, an approach based on shared assumptions by psychiatrists and Christians. Yet I am fully aware that what I suggest is nothing more than a starting point, a common table at which both psychiatrists and Christians can sit. Who knows where the conversation may lead? My only prediction is that the conversation, if it truly addresses the vacuum I perceive, will be difficult and threatening. The conversation will draw both psychiatrists and Christians out of their comfort zones. Debate will be inevitable, but it need not be vitriolic. Cultures will clash, but these clashes need not lead to cultural wars.

Why should we risk a conversation and perhaps place psychiatry and Christianity at odds with one another in the midst of our present accommodation? Because the accommodation does not work! Real people suffering severe emotional problems are not being helped as well as they could be helped. We may be treating mental illness, but we are not caring for persons in their faith communities. I believe we can gain from a conversation—gain insight for ourselves and gain quality care for those who suffer. The risk is necessary; the vulnerability must be tolerated. I do not believe any of us will find a comfortable yet honest integration. But failure to reach ultimate integration will be more than compensated by an increased sensitivity to persons who suffer severe emotional problems.

6

The Care of Souls & Minds

Making Conversation Between Psychiatry & Christianity

A*t a meeting of psychiatrists inter-*
ested in the interface between psychiatry and Christianity, Armand Nicholi
from Harvard University described a most interesting project. Nicholi
teaches an undergraduate seminar entitled "Two World Views." In this
seminar he requires students to read selected writings of Freud—*Civilization and Its Discontents, Totem and Taboo* and *Moses and Monotheism*—
which describe Freud's worldview. He also requires students to read
selected writings of the literary critic and converted Christian C. S. Lewis,
such as *Mere Christianity, Miracles* and *The Problem of Pain.*[1] Participants
in the seminar are a mixture of Christians, persons of other faith persuasions
and persons who profess no faith. The contrasting worldviews of Freud and
Lewis stimulate a lively, at times heated, but rarely threatening conversation
and debate among these students. Nicholi showed a videotape of one of the
seminar sessions, an inspiring interchange among students from most
diverse backgrounds.

I asked Nicholi if he believed such a interchange would be possible
among a group of practicing psychiatrists with such diverse backgrounds.

We agreed it would be difficult. Flexibility of thought and willingness to risk statements of belief, whatever that belief may be, often become ossified as we mature. In addition, we accumulate much baggage during our careers as doctors first and psychiatrists later, baggage that renders discussion of one's worldview much more complex. I suspect the same could be said about mature Christian theologians. The psychiatrists sitting around that table envied the freedom, spontaneity and energy of the students in the videotape. Every student demonstrated a courage to speak out and risk a frontal attack on her or his worldview. No student accepted either Freud's or Lewis's worldview uncritically. The discussion was complex, but not to the point that open discussion was muted.

An Integrated Approach
How do we begin a meaningful conversation between psychiatry and Christianity? The previous conversation soured and then disappeared, I believe, because of an excess of ideology, a lack of theory and, frankly, a lack of courage on both sides. Psychiatrists may shudder at the thought that our specialty is plagued with ideology today. Neuropsychiatrists were quick to criticize the unscientific ideology of psychoanalysis at midcentury. In fact, it was this critique of psychoanalysis that ushered in the empirical approach to classification which culminated in the production of DSM-III in 1980 and the subsequent decline of psychoanalysis as an accepted form of therapy (see chapter two). The explicit ideology of psychoanalysis, however, has been replaced by the implicit ideology of neuropsychiatry today. In my view, the ideology that undergirds neuropsychiatry is as grounded in the ideology of social science of the nineteenth century and faith in the scientific method as was the ideology of psychoanalysis.

Some may question whether psychiatry is a medical specialty grounded in social science as opposed to physical science. As long as we work with people who live in communities and express their mental illnesses in language, we will be at least as grounded in social science as we are grounded in molecules. The scientific method undergirds both the physical and the social sciences. In actuality, they cross-fertilize each other.

What was the ideology that dominated the social sciences during the nineteenth century? I believe that there is no one predominant ideology across the social sciences today, but this was not always the case. Positivism, the belief that the "natural" sciences provide the only valid model for all human knowledge, ruled the social sciences during the nineteenth century. Objectivity was "out there," beyond human beings. To be value-free was the only way to be scientific.[2] This ideology now dominates psychiatry perhaps more than it dominates nuclear physics. Physicists learned early in the twentieth century that the very process of observing subatomic phenomena disturbs those phenomena. That is, observation is by definition biased—hence the uncertainty principle of Werner Heisenberg. Modern psychiatrists, in contrast, have an implicit confidence in their ability to observe both molecules and behavior without bias; they believe their relationship to what they observe does not interfere with the observation.

This faith in objectivity, this positivism among neuropsychiatrists, perhaps emerged as a reaction to the perceived unscientific claims of psychoanalysis. During the late 1960s and early 1970s psychoanalysis was at times an embarrassment to psychiatrists. When I interacted with medical colleagues from other specialties while in training, I felt like a used-car salesman dealing a second-rate, unproven and frequently ineffective product among the busy, high-tech internists and surgeons. I could gain their attention only when I could do something that worked and worked quickly. Prescribing medications or electroconvulsive therapy to the severely depressed did work and was quick enough. These therapies were proven effective by the scientific method.

I rejoined medicine as I practiced neuropsychiatry. So did my fellow psychiatrists. One respected older colleague proclaimed at an early meeting of the American College of Neuropsychopharmacology (ACNP) during this era that "psychiatry *is* and *only is* biological psychiatry." The ACNP soon eclipsed the American Psychoanalytic Association and became, I believe, the premier gathering of psychiatrists during the 1980s. New discoveries in neurobiology and psychopharmacology grew at a geometric rate.

Unfortunately, theory has lagged behind discovery. Some psychiatrists, such as Leston Havens and Ed Hundert, have attempted to integrate philosophy, psychiatry and neuroscience, but few modern psychiatrists read their works. The field has progressed at too rapid a pace to be encumbered by theory, since today's theory may be rendered obsolete by tomorrow's discovery. Or perhaps a struggle with theory takes us out of our comfort zone. Regardless, even as today's psychiatrists may sense a need for deeper theoretical foundations to understand the massive data that are emerging from neurobiology, they do not appear to know where to begin. We have not been educated to think about theory. We have rather been trained to assimilate data and follow prescribed algorithms.

Christian theologians and counselors are no different. The study of religion has become highly specialized. In theology, once considered equivalent to developing a comprehensive theory, or a systematic theology, comprehensive efforts to integrate have diminished. Paul Tillich did not hesitate to write a systematic (and comprehensive) theology (not to mention a review of art and culture).[3] My colleagues at Duke's Divinity School admit, however, that the field has not produced a Niebuhr or a Tillich in many years. This should not surprise us. Both psychiatry and Christianity must work from a much more complex, sizable and confusing knowledge base. A comprehensive theory, a worldview, is not nearly so easy to produce and defend. In fact those who today would be so presumptuous as to propose a comprehensive theory would likely be ignored or ridiculed. Yet can we engage in meaningful conversation without theory?

A comment by the anthropologist Clifford Geertz in 1973, regarding anthropological work on religion, makes this point:

Two characteristics of anthropological work on religion accomplished since the second world war strike me as curious when such work is placed against that carried out just before and just after the first. One is that it has made no theoretical advances of major importance. It is living off the conceptual capital of its ancestors, adding very little, save a certain empirical enrichment, to it. The second is that it draws what concepts it does use from a very narrowly defined intellectual tradition. . . . Virtually no one even thinks of looking elsewhere—to philosophy, history, law, literature, or the "harder" sciences . . . for analytical ideas. And it occurs to me also that these two curious characteristics are not unrelated.[4]

I believe that few major theoretical advances to understanding the interface between Christianity and psychiatry have been made during the past twenty-five years. In contrast, some advances have been made in the integration of philosophy, psychiatry and neuroscience, advances that are most relevant to the conversation between psychiatry and Christianity.

Edward Hundert, for example, has provided us with a masterful synthesis, a "synthetic analysis," of these three areas of inquiry.[5] Taking G. W. F. Hegel's dialectic and Immanuel Kant's categories as a starting point, Hundert argues for an ontology (a science of the existence of humankind) and a phenomenology (the study of living experience). He ties the Hegelian phenomenology of spirit or the becoming of knowledge to Jean Piaget's seminal observations of the child's progressive construction of reality and how that construction can go astray in mental illness. Then he continues his synthesis of these three diverse areas of inquiry by exploring our current knowledge of how the brain and its receptors of the external events shape and are shaped by a dynamic interaction, an interaction that philosophically reaches back to antiquity and was formulated for the modern era by Kant.

The key concept for Hundert is "intersubjectivity," recognizing the dynamic and subjective nature of the growth of and development of persons in relation to others. Yet theologians and psychiatrists have neglected to advance our understanding of the critical interface between neuropsychiatry and religion, perhaps the most important intersubjective relationship of all. Hundert stops short of exploring this interface, yet perhaps provides an avenue for exploration via the synthesis of philosophy and neuropsychiatry through psychiatry.

I believe paradigms that currently drive empirical work by both psychiatrists and Christian counselors draw on narrow and poorly recognized intellectual traditions that do not step back to the philosophical, much less the theological. The traditions that have evolved have been undergirded by either implicit theories such as those which undergird evolutionary biology or ideologies that are not so much carefully thought through as loudly proclaimed. In this book I have tried to describe those traditions and demonstrate to what extent they structure the writings of psychiatrists and Christian counselors.

Psychiatry and Christianity, I believe, can break from their current narrow paradigms through a meaningful, if at times heated, conversation and debate. Perhaps I will be accused of being overly optimistic when I suggest that we can sit at the same table as do those Harvard undergraduates, exploring the really tough questions and opening ourselves to a frontal attack on our personal as well as professional worldviews. Such a conversation will surely lead to confrontations that most of us can easily avoid by playing out our roles within our present comfortable confines. A challenge to our implicit theories about emotional suffering, which we hold tightly whether we have thought them through carefully or not, will both awaken our minds and stimulate our souls. Some of the courage found in the undergraduate student remains in each of us. I believe we will join the conversation if we know where to begin.

What elements are necessary for this conversation? A set theory is not necessary as a point of departure, but a desire to develop a more comprehensive theory *is* necessary. Both psychiatrists and Christian theologians/counselors must be willing to expand their theoretical as well as their empirical boundaries. I suggest the following. First, some assumptions must be shared by both psychiatrists and Christian theologians/counselors. If not, the conversation will quickly derail into an irreconcilable conflict. Second, given these assumptions, psychiatrists and Christians should begin meaningful conversations through the process of asking questions about real persons in real communities as well as questions about advances in the neurosciences, as I have described in chapter one. These conversations do not guarantee better accommodation or integration. They will, however, assure a more honest assessment of each field of inquiry and deeper self-assessment among those persons at the interface, whether they are psychiatrists, Christian counselors or patients. If we come to the table of conversation and debate after having worked with persons experiencing emotional pain, we will leave the table more sober, better informed and, I believe, more effective in caring for these persons.

I outline below what I believe to be assumptions that must be shared by psychiatrists and Christian theologians/counselors for a meaningful conversation to emerge. I am not so naive as to think all psychiatrists and Christian theological counselors are willing to engage in this conversation. Both psychiatry and Christianity, especially evangelical Christianity, are too pluralistic and fragmented to universally agree even on the assumptions necessary for beginning a conversation. Yet many persons within psychiatry and Christianity do share the assumptions I believe necessary for conversation. Those who engage the conversation need not be Christians who accept the mechanistic philosophy that underlies certain psychiatric therapies, nor need they be psychiatrists who accept the validity of the Christian faith. They only must be at the table, willing to engage in open and honest discussion and debate.

I also believe the conversation should occur at multiple levels. Given the shared areas of concern and activity, institutional psychiatry and the church should pursue dialogues as exemplified by the visit of the president of the American Psychiatric Association to the Vatican. These public overtures will not in themselves ensure meaningful dialogue. They will, however, provide a public display of the removal of perceived barriers, which in turn will open the opportunity for dialogue. Individual practitioners of psychiatry and members of the Christian community must attempt a dialogue, even if they find themselves speaking on different planes or at cross-purposes. At the least, both psychiatrists and Christians can better recognize the language, not to mention the assumptions, of the other. Finally, psychiatrists who are Christian must carry on an internal dialogue and avoid the temptation to compartmentalize their lives. What are the shared assumptions that render conversation possible?

Shared Assumptions

Humankind exists in a state of striving for meaning. I believe all human beings experience strivings. The debate over the nature of these strivings is significant, and a consensus regarding their origins is not necessary for a conversation between psychiatry and Christianity. Some suggest that strivings simply play a role in the maintenance of essential psychic conditions—that is, they maintain homeostasis.[6] Others suggest that these strivings can be reduced to simple and specific explanations. For example, we strive for food because of our specific need of nourishment, or we strive to know God because there is a God. Jean-Jacques Rousseau, for example, believed strivings can be reduced to a primary striving for food and shelter, with other strivings being elaborations of such primary strivings.[7] Anselm articulated the ontological argument for the existence of God—that there must be a God because we recognize something than which nothing greater can be conceived.[8]

The traditional Freudian explanation for spiritual strivings leaves little room for factors beyond the wishful person. Wish fulfillment, specifically fulfillment of the wish for the powerful lost father, is a necessary and sufficient reason for the existence of God in the mind of humankind. The ontological argument, meanwhile, leaves little room for distortions of this striving, or for its integration with others that may occur during the midst of a severe emotional problem. Because there is a God, persons naturally seek the nature of that true God. Both Anselm's and Freud's explanations neglect study of the phenomena of spiritual and social strivings, phenomena that are observable to anyone studying humankind. I believe strivings, especially strivings for value, meaning and relationship, are more primary than many thinkers are willing to accept.

When I first entered psychiatry, I was attracted to the writings of the social psychiatrist Alexander Leighton. He recognized these strivings and attempted to place them within a comprehensive theory that did not attempt to explain their origins (whether the striving was based on a need for nourishment or for God) but rather to understand the context of these strivings. At that point I knew little about psychiatric illness, yet I was wary of the reductionistic ideologies of both psychoanalytic psychiatry and fundamentalist Christianity. Leighton provided me with a welcome opening for a conversation between psychiatry and Christianity (though this was not the primary goal of his work).

Leighton described these strivings as sentiments, a union of thought and feeling dependent on a combination of basic urges and conscious factors.[9] He suggested that sentiments must be considered within the context of an individual's life story, having evolved during the course of growth and experience as well as progressively differentiating from basic instincts and from each other. The essential striving sentiments, according to Leighton, are

- ☐ physical security
- ☐ sexual satisfaction
- ☐ the expression of hostility
- ☐ the expression of love
- ☐ the securing of love
- ☐ the securing of recognition
- ☐ the expression of spontaneity (called variously positive force, creativity, volition)
- ☐ the securing and maintaining of membership in a definite human group
- ☐ a sense of belonging to a moral order and being right in what one does, being in and of a system of values[10]

Some will take issue with Leighton's list of sentiments, especially striving for moral order. Empirically, however, few can argue that humankind expresses this sentiment. Ed Hundert, for example, in *Lessons from an Optical Illusion: On Nature and Nurture, Knowledge and Values,* accepts moral order yet places it in an evolutionary-biology context.[11] Alasdair MacIntyre, in *After Virtue,* has argued that even though we have lost our comprehension (both theoretical and practical) of morality, we have not lost a concern for meaning within individuals or in subcultures, nor the inherent drive for morality within the individual.[12] Christians view the origins of a moral order (an aspect of spirituality, if you will) as deriving from a transcendent source. For the purposes of conversation between psychiatry and Christianity, it is not necessary that the origin of this sentiment be agreed on, but only that the sentiment be recognized.

Leighton's list of striving sentiments is grounded in a particular perspective of communal relationship of which the striving for moral order is only one aspect. He therefore brings me full circle to where I began my argument. Psychiatry is about soul, if by soul we mean the person in relationship with her or his perceived God and others. To understand emotional suffering, both psychiatrist and Christian must recognize persons in this context.

Emotional suffering must be understood from the perspective of the person suffering. Psychiatrists tend to diagnose psychiatric disorders; Christian counselors tend to identify maladaptive coping strategies based on deviance from prescribed adaptive behaviors derived from Scripture.

From the perspective of persons experiencing emotional pain, however, psychiatric disorder and maladaptive coping merge. These persons suffer. They suffer emotional pain and disordered behavior, yet to them the two are one and the same. Barbara, Jason (chapter one) and many others view their problems differently from most psychiatrists. For those persons embedded in the Christian tradition, emotional pain cannot be disentangled from one's relationship to God, which is frequently perceived as severely strained in the midst of emotional pain. God, as often as not, is viewed as the enemy, not a support, in the midst of suffering.

Persons in deep suffering view their pain differently from the typical Christian counselor who calls on God to heal the pain. The suffering are not convinced that God will heal what he has visited upon them. Both psychiatrists and Christians must understand emotional suffering from the perspective of the person. By recognizing and empathizing with suffering, the psychiatrist and the Christian counselor begin the relationship with the person which can lead to healing.

Emotional suffering occurs within a person's life history. No personal experience, or thought for that matter, can be isolated from the life history of the person. Betty's response to relief of symptoms (see chapter one) is in large part determined by her history of helping and being helped. Each individual is a continuous emergence from conception to death, influenced by both hereditary disposition and experiences with the physical and social environment. In other words, we cannot understand the person if we do not recognize that he or she is the product of a previous life story as it interacts with the current situation.[13]

Religious beliefs and actions, as well as emotional suffering, are woven within the fabric of one's life history. Much of what we have learned through the psychological sciences directly informs us about the life history of the person. Studies of memory, personality development, intellectual and social growth, and critical transitions in life (such as adolescence) contribute to our understanding of life history. As psychiatrists or Christian counselors, we are usually privy to only a brief window of that history and therefore may fail to recognize the need for the person to integrate emotional suffering within her or his life story. The significance of the life story, especially a person's spiritual story, is critical to the conversation between psychiatrists and Christian theologians and counselors.

Personal histories evolve within the context of relationships. The life history of an individual evolves within the context of a relationship. Emphasis on individualism in American society tends to blunt our recognition of the impact of the sociocultural environment on growth and development. Human beings are intimately connected to many self-integrating units, based on patterns of interpersonal relations, communications, symbols and mores. The "culture" or "community" in which persons live out their life histories is divided into overlapping subcultures, such as family, neighborhood, workplace and religious community. Christian tradition and the local church are key components of that sociocultural environment for millions of Americans—and people from other parts of the world as well.

The American evangelical community has evolved rapidly in recent years. Any mental health professional who treats evangelical Christians would do well to understand that evolution. Evangelicals have developed their own subculture in the midst of the diverse American culture. Even as evangelicals fight in the political arena against abortion and for prayer in public schools, they have developed a media empire with television and radio stations (not just programs), publications and support groups. They have developed a network of private schools, from kindergarten to college. Many evangelical families are now choosing to home school. They have increasingly withdrawn from secular society. The emergence of the Christian counseling industry, parallel to but interacting rarely with secular psychology and psychiatry, is but part of a larger separatist movement among evangelicals. Even as evangelicals tend to withdraw, however, they shape relationships within American society by their large numbers and their political influence.

Psychology and psychiatry shape relationships within the sociocultural environment as well. Martin Gross describes American society as

the most anxious, emotionally insecure and analyzed population in the history of man, the citizens of the contemporary psychological society. It [the psychological society] is also about that society's practitioners, the psychiatrist and psychologist who have built an elaborate professional structure to cater to our emotional needs. . . . Its citizen is a new model of western man, one who is dependent on others for guidance as to what is real or false.[14]

When Gross published his book *The Psychological Society* in 1978, he scarcely anticipated the emergence of neuropsychiatry and instead focused on the influence of psychotherapy. Today secular psychotherapy of all varieties is under siege. Health maintenance organizations (HMOs) and managed care companies refuse to pay for services that are not "proven effective." For psychotherapy, this usually translates into ten or fewer sessions provided per year, with a sizable copay (frequently 50 percent) required from the patient. Though some possess the resources to go outside the system, many others who would have sought and received psychotherapy in the past from psychiatrists no longer do so. By default, the prescription of a psychotherapeutic medication coupled with a few visits for medication checks has become the norm for treating severe emotional suffering. We still live in a psychological society, yet neuropsychiatry now rules, and it ignores or devalues the role of relationships, the role of soul, in emotional suffering.

To recognize the influence of evangelical Christianity and neuropsychiatry on society is not enough. The psychiatrist must study the culture of the evangelical Christian and attempt to empathize with as well as understand it. The Christian must recognize and empathize with psychiatry, especially a psychiatry pressured toward quick, individualistic therapies within our rapidly evolving health care system. Though current sociocultural movements are complex and confusing, they are powerful forces that shape how psychiatrists and Christians think and act.

The care and cure of the emotional suffering are shared within a society. No psychiatric disorder is the exclusive province of a psychiatrist. No experience of profound existential depression is the exclusive province of the church. To suggest that the psychiatrist and the church must work together in order to provide comprehensive care for persons with severe emotional problems is to understate the issue. The schizophrenic woman who belongs to a community of Christians, such as Barbara (chapter one), will necessarily be cared for by that community, whether that care is effective or ineffective. That same woman, in American society, almost inevitably will be receiving professional mental health care and probably medications. The church and the psychiatrist are not alone, however, in caring for the schizophrenic woman. Federal and state governments provide certain benefits to the psychiatrically impaired, such as social security benefits because of disability.

Society also restricts these persons, in that some behaviors will not be tolerated (behaviors dangerous to self and others); these behaviors may lead to institutionalization or isolation from society. As the ranks of the homeless are filled with persons with schizophrenia, ever more social programs and agencies become involved with persons suffering this disorder. The evangelical church is among the many groups attempting to minister to the homeless, yet frustrated in its efforts because it doesn't understand mental illness. Psychiatrists and Christian theologians/counselors must appreciate their mutual roles in caring for persons suffering emotional problems and inform one another.

Theory cannot lag far behind practice in the care of souls. Freud was correct when he suggested that psychological processes and religious beliefs/behaviors are inevitably interwoven. Foucault was correct when he suggested that mental illness cannot be extracted objectively from the context of a society in which persons are labeled as either mentally healthy or mentally ill. Humankind by nature seeks to classify and explain the phenomena, both psychological and religious, that it observes. Our actions are based on explicit or implicit theories. Both psychiatry and Christianity are built on a set of concepts plus their interrelationships.

Concepts of importance to the conversation between psychiatry and Christianity are numerous but include "emotional suffering," "moral sentiments," "life history" and "soul." I have referred to these concepts throughout this book, but I have not attempted to set forth a theory that integrates these concepts, nor have I stated hypotheses that might derive from such a theory. As noted earlier, to propose such a theory is not the purpose of this book. Nevertheless, the reader must not assume that I take a theoretical approach to what I see, hear, feel and believe. I am at work on theory constantly. I think through relationships, I draw diagrams, I attempt my own definitions of concepts, all in the service of explaining emotional pain such as experienced by someone who is severely depressed.

Do not expect psychiatrists or Christians to care for the emotionally suffering without proposing theories about the phenomena they observe. These theories may not be overt, and they rarely crystallize, but they *will* emerge, evolve and come into conflict if the minds of practitioners are alive. Discussions of these theoretical conflicts strengthen our understanding and our ability to care effectively for persons suffering emotionally. Mindless, a theoretical psychiatry and Christianity cannot survive.

Islands of community can be found in the sea of diversity. No one can reasonably argue that America is a unified culture, either a Christian nation or a secular society. Cultural wars, which James Davison Hunter suggests are a struggle to define America for different subcultures, are perhaps the result of a desire to reestablish a culture that at one time was perceived to be more unified and now has become more diverse.[15] Yet subcultures do not simply line up left versus right, liberal versus conservative or secular versus religious. We are a most diverse society.

Within this cultural diversity there exist islands of unity. At times groups that seem to be unified in fact consist of multiple cultures that align only for short periods behind some common cause, such as the alignment of Christian fundamentalists, Orthodox Jews and conservative Catholics in the battle against their perceived counterparts for control of American culture.[16] More often, and for longer periods of time, smaller groups with common values align themselves.

Theologians Stanley Hauerwas and William Willimon, in their book *Resident Aliens,* explore the so-called alien status of Christians in the secular West and suggest that accepting the identity of resident aliens will provide Christians with a framework for relating to and supporting one another. They quote the apostle Paul, "Our citizenship is in heaven" (Phil 3:20), and propose the concept of the Christian community as a colony. "A colony is a beach head, an outpost, an island of one culture in the middle of another."[17]

Hauerwas and Willimon carry this argument a step further. The church, as a colony among aliens, is a place where the values of home are reiterated and passed on to the young, a place where the distinctive language and lifestyle of the resident aliens are lovingly nurtured and reinforced. . . . To be resident but alien is a formula for loneliness that few of us can sustain. Indeed, it is almost impossible to minister alone because our loneliness can too quickly turn into self-righteousness or self-hate. Christians can only survive by supporting one another through the countless small acts through which we tell one another we are not alone, that God is with us. Friendship is not, therefore, accidental to Christian life.[18]

For a conversation between psychiatry and Christianity to be meaningful, psychiatrists must recognize not only the actual but the potential strength of Christian culture, and especially individual Christian communities. The authority and influence of the local church has declined over the past few years among evangelicals, but the church remains an important institution. The church may well become more influential in the future if Christians recognize that they are truly a minority in a diverse society and that political action will not return society to the perceived "one nation under God" of past generations.

Christians, in like manner, must recognize the community, or at least the need for community, among psychiatrists. Granted, it is difficult to find unity among psychiatrists, or even a desire for unity. Psychiatrists, however, are in many ways aliens among health care professionals. At present the trend in psychiatry is to blur boundaries between psychiatry and the remainder of medicine, as has been discussed throughout this book. The emphasis on neuropsychiatry and the empirical medical model are examples of this return to mainstream medicine. I suspect, however, that this trend will not persist. There is enough unique about the care of the mentally ill and the characteristics of the individuals who choose to care for them that psychiatrists will again reclaim their communal boundaries.

Psychiatry has flourished during times when its identity has been distinct. At the very time that the neurosciences have exploded and psychiatry has become a more accepted specialty, the numbers of persons seeking training in psychiatry have decreased. Many factors contribute to this decline of interest in psychiatry, such as the emphasis on primary care, but I believe that a sense of distinctiveness within community, similar to that experienced by psychiatrists during Freud's era, may reemerge to offset this decline. Christians must recognize the importance and need for community among psychiatrists. Treating the mentally ill, the "insane," has always been a lonely task. Just as the psychiatrist cannot fully understand and converse with the emotionally suffering Christian without an appreciation of the faith community, evangelical Christians cannot understand and converse with a psychiatrist unless they appreciate the psychiatric community.

A prime unifying factor among psychiatrists during the early years of the twentieth century was a moral unity based on the ethical (though perhaps not religious) principles of Freud. With the fall of psychoanalysis, the moral unity of psychiatry has been replaced by a moral diversity, perhaps even a moral chaos. Alasdair MacIntyre is generally pessimistic about the current moral chaos, which he describes as a new Dark Ages, in our society as a whole. Nevertheless, he believes there is an opportunity, even a necessity, for reinstating "local forms of community in which civility and the intellectual and moral life can be sustained through the new dark ages."[19]

MacIntyre believes our society can go even further. He suggests that rival and incompatible positions on moral issues can be addressed, if not resolved, when we recognize that different positions are not totally isolated but are rooted in different traditions of justification. If those living moral traditions are but comprehended, "the problem of diversity is not abandoned, but transformed in a way that renders it amenable of solution."[20] MacIntyre could easily be writing about modern psychiatry. Psychiatry is ultimately about caring for persons who experience perhaps the most devastating pains that plague humankind, emotional pains. Rededication to this moral task, I believe, is the call to community among psychiatrists.

James Davison Hunter, however, believes finding agreement within the disagreement and diversity of society will require more of us.[21] Though he doesn't speak directly to psychiatrists, Hunter suggests a series of practical steps that, if applied by psychiatrists to psychiatry, could reestablish the professional community. First, the environment of public discourse must change. Specifically, the reinstitution of genuine debate would be most useful, for isolated extremist rhetoric is difficult to maintain in a discursive environment. Some years ago this type of debate was instituted as a regular feature during the annual meeting of the American Psychiatric Association. In my opinion those debates have shed much light on many conflicts in psychiatry, such as the change from the more theoretical, psychoanalytically based nomenclature of DSM-II to the more empirical, neuropsychiatric nomenclature of DSM-III (see chapter three).

Second, Hunter proposes that all factions reject the impulse toward public quiescence. He suggests that people in the middle of a debate tend to refrain from speaking up due to excessive outpouring of rhetoric from the extremes. Few psychiatrists are purely mechanistic and few are purely theistic in their philosophy. These middle-ground practitioners and academicians must join the conversation if true community is to be reestablished within the profession

Third, Hunter suggests that society must recognize the sacred within different subcultures. By "sacred" he means the nonnegotiable, that which defines the limits of a subculture. If psychiatrists are to build community, the profession must recognize the nonnegotiables of its diverse members. For years psychiatry was perceived as a profession that did not recognize that which is sacred to the conservative, evangelical Christian. As Christians have felt more comfortable in the profession, other diverse groups have felt more comfortable as well, such as Muslims, African-Americans, women and homosexuals. The profession is no longer an exclusive club of secular white males. Yet the acceptance of diverse groups has not been accompanied by a parallel move toward respect for that diversity. For example, can psychiatry respect conservative Christians and the gay community simultaneously? Perhaps not, but there has been too little effort to establish community across diverse nonnegotiables. I believe that if the profession is to survive, these respective nonnegotiables must be identified and acknowledged by the profession. I also believe commonalities essential to the profession can be found within diversity.

Finally, Hunter suggests that groups must recognize the inherent weaknesses, even dangers, in their own moral commitment. Here psychiatry (as well as evangelical Christianity) has much work to do. Many psychiatrists have not considered the moral implications of modern neuropsychiatry.

They assume that it is value-free, much as the psychoanalytic community in years past expounded a value-free psychiatry while degrading the values and morals of conservative Christians and other faith traditions (such as Orthodox Judaism and Islam).

Of course these same principles apply to evangelical Christianity, although there is a qualitative difference between psychiatry and Christianity when they do come to the table to converse. Psychiatrists do not perceive their communal identity to the extent that Christians perceive their communal identity. Identity is ultimately grounded in beliefs and values, not facts. Christians, despite their diversity, recognize that their identity is based in a faith tradition. Psychiatrists, in contrast, are not nearly as certain about their identity, for they rarely discuss the values on which their practices are based.

A long tradition among critics of psychiatry, such as Foucault (see chapter three), suggests that psychiatry is a willing instrument by which society controls persons with behavior that deviates from societal norms. Psychiatry may be guilty of being such an instrument at the turn of the millennium, but if so, it does not do so knowingly. Psychiatrists rarely address the larger societal implications of their actions because they are oriented toward individuals, especially in the 1990s. Not since the mental health movement of the 1950s and 1960s has psychiatry cast its eyes seriously on society as a whole.

In contrast, Christianity is by its nature interested in the community. Today evangelical Christianity is taking political steps to shape the community at large. I believe these steps are ill-advised and ultimately damaging to the church. Yet evangelical Christianity takes these steps with the conviction that they will be successful.

Christianity is not alone in expressing concern about the moral status of society. Psychiatry as a profession has, in the past, expressed its concerns about the ills of society as well. The social psychiatrists of the 1950s and 1960s, grounded in psychoanalysis and sociology/anthropology, focused on society's ills. Their prescription for society was value-driven, encouraging openness, mutual support and special support for those experiencing emotional suffering. Such communal expressions of social concern and values could emerge again among psychiatrists.

In any case, if conversation is to be meaningful, Christianity must understand the underlying values, not just the facts, that drive psychiatry.

The Journey Has Barely Begun

The care and cure of souls is not new. Yet the striving for emotional and physical well-being has not always been as segregated as it tends to be in modern society. In ancient societies the healer of the body and the healer of the soul were one and the same, such as the shaman among Native Americans or the wise man among the Hebrews.[22] Even during the early years of psychiatry as a medical specialty, a conversation between Christianity and psychiatry scarcely existed. When the conversation began it was dominated by the metaphor of the Freud versus God debate. That energizing debate is now ended.

Other factors now dominate our discourse about the care of emotional suffering. I have concentrated in this book on my concerns about neuropsychiatry and commonsense Christian counseling. Yet the cost of health care has emerged as the ultimate determinant of care of those suffering emotionally. Persons who suffer, such as Jason, can all too easily be ignored. The real need for conversation thus has scarcely begun. At the least, conversation and debate will keep the focus on individuals who suffer. At best, we will learn to care for them as real persons and value their minds and souls as much as we value our own.

I believe it is fitting to end this book with yet another story of my relationship with a Christian who experienced emotional suffering. This story did not leave me questioning as do the stories in chapter one. It provides me with confidence that we *can* explore the interface between psychiatry and Christianity and reclaim the soul of psychiatry and the mind of evangelical Christianity.

Richard's Long Journey

I first became acquainted with Richard over twenty years ago, when he was fifty-eight years old. He brought his son Tom for treatment, and I agreed to accept Tom as a patient. Tom was twenty-eight years old at the time and had been hospitalized on many occasions for secondary to acute symptoms of schizophrenia. Nevertheless, Tom had maintained regular employment between hospitalizations as a systems manager for mainframe computers.

My interaction with Richard initially was through brief visits with him, as he always accompanied Tom to his three-month medication checkups. About a year after I undertook Tom's care, Tom experienced an acute psychotic episode. He was hospitalized for three weeks, and convincing him to take his medication was difficult. Richard became my best ally in working with Tom, and I appreciated much better Richard's support of his son. It was Richard's constant monitoring and assistance that permitted Tom to function as well as he did.

Yet Richard's attention was not directed to Tom alone. He was a successful lawyer in a small North Carolina town and was known and respected for accepting difficult cases and defending the underdog. Richard was also a member of the board of deacons at the local Baptist church and a member of the school board. His energy was exceptional for his age (or any age for that matter). The more I came to know Richard, the more I learned of his tireless efforts to help others. He was most knowledgeable about psychiatric illness, given his many years facilitating Tom's care, and recognized the need for support groups to assist family members caring for persons with severe emotional suffering. He initiated a regional chapter of the National Association for the Mentally Ill (NAMI).

Five years after I became acquainted with Richard, his wife, Kay, developed Alzheimer's disease. Richard retired from his law practice and became her primary caretaker. Kay proved to be afflicted with a variety of Alzheimer's that progresses rapidly, and her mental and physical abilities declined precipitously over the next four years. Richard somehow managed to care for her with minimal assistance at home until six months prior to her death (when she was placed in a nursing home). During Kay's illness Richard maintained his supportive relationship with Tom. Tom himself was hospitalized twice during his mother's illness, but overall functioned somewhat better than he had prior to her illness. He became more involved in the church where Richard was a deacon and joined a softball team (where he found that he had talent as a pitcher). Tom also dated frequently, though he expressed no interest in getting married. Richard was delighted with the progressive independence Tom exhibited.

During Kay's illness, however, Richard first asked me to consult with him about his own problems. Caretaking responsibilities coupled with his concern about Tom's future had precipitated a moderately severe depression. Despite the severity of his symptoms (he had difficulty sleeping, a poor appetite with a ten-pound weight loss, difficulty concentrating and a feeling that everything he did was an effort), Richard rarely missed a day of his caretaking activities, and Tom, like Richard's close friends, did not recognize that Richard was suffering emotionally. Richard felt guilty about becoming depressed and especially about wishing that Kay would not live much longer. He believed, perhaps, that God was testing him and he was failing the test.

In the past, Richard believed, every challenge God placed before him had been met with success, whether it was caring for Tom or defending an unpopular client in his law practice. Nevertheless, Richard understood the biological nature of severe depression, recognized that he was experiencing more stress than ever before, and believed that he needed treatment with an antidepressant medication.

I agreed with him and prescribed the antidepressant nortriptyline. He responded well, with virtually all the symptoms disappearing within three months, remained on the medication for six months and then was able to discontinue its use.

Following Kay's death, Richard (sixty-seven years old at the time) began volunteer work at the local high school, first as a support person in the office and later as an informal counselor and tutor for kids who needed individual attention. He loved his work, and he was loved for his work. He also became more involved with his church, visiting lonely persons who could not leave their homes due to illness. In his words, Richard wished to be "an inspiration and encouragement to others." He experienced periodic episodes of depression over the following eight years, none as severe as the first and all responding to a brief course of nortriptyline. During these episodes I did not feel a need to engage Richard in any type of psychotherapy beyond simple support.

When Richard was seventy-six, he experienced a severe heart attack that resulted in permanent damage to much of his heart. Few thought he would survive, but he did. Nevertheless, Richard did not recover his physical functioning, and over the following year Tom was forced to become Richard's caretaker, performing most tasks around the house, such as cooking and shopping. Tom seemed to thrive in his new role of caretaker and managed these tasks well while maintaining his job and other outside activities.

Richard told me, "I could not be more proud of Tom. I now believe that when I am gone, Tom will be able to care for himself." Richard also was overwhelmed with the support and attention he received from his church and community. The year following his heart attack was filled with banquets in his honor and awards for lifetime service to the community.

Richard, however, was far from happy. He became severely depressed three months following the heart attack, a depression that "felt different" from the episodes of depression he had experienced in the past. Nortriptyline relieved his sleep but did not relieve his profound sadness and unexpected anger. Richard said, "I should be able to manage this illness, but I can't." First he asked that we try some of the new antidepressants, such as Prozac, Zoloft and Paxil. None relieved his symptoms, and each produced side effects that further complicated his depression. We returned to nortriptyline as the best antidepressant under the circumstances.

Both Richard and I became discouraged. One day, during an office visit, Richard said, "I am having a fight with God."

I asked him to explain what he meant, and he responded, "I have always been in control. I have been the caretaker, I have been the 'hand of God.' Now God has taken his hand away from me. It's more than that, though. I thought I understood my relationship with God, yet now I feel isolated from both God and the people around me.

"Don't get me wrong. My friends have been as supportive as I could ask. Yet they knew the old Richard, the strong Richard. They knew the Richard who had a confidence in God and in himself that wouldn't quit, yet that confidence is waning. What would happen if I told them that I was having a fight with God, that God had let me down and I didn't like it? What would happen if they knew that I shout at him and question his judgment? All I have done in the name of God and for the community would be for naught. So here I am, alone yet surrounded by others, apparently blessed by a loving God but feeling cursed by the 'Master of the universe,' who has decided to upset at the end of my life the entire meaning of my life."

At one level, I had no difficulty diagnosing Richard's problem. He suffered a treatment-resistant depression, not uncommon following a severe physical illness. In addition, Richard had every reason to feel depressed, despite all he said about his "blessings." He had been a helper and in control of his own life throughout his adult life and had accomplished much. One of Richard's worst fears must have been that he would be a burden on the very people to whom he had dedicated his life in caretaking and support. Yet I believe his worst fear was the perception that his relationship with God—that he was the hand or instrument of God—would be challenged.

Richard knew why he was depressed and angry as well as I. How was I to help him?

My traditional tools as a psychiatrist were rendered useless. Medications weren't getting the job done. Commonsense therapy would have fallen flat. For example, I could have told Richard he had earned the right to relax and accept help from others. Not only would that advice have fallen on deaf ears, but Richard would have recognized that I did not really know him after all the years we had worked together. Psychoanalytic interpretations would have been equally useless. I could have asked Richard to tell me about his anger with God, perhaps associating that anger with his projection of helplessness in the presence of a harsh father, as his father had indeed been. Yet Richard would not have accepted the association of his present anger with God and anger with his father in the past. God was a problem for Richard in the here and now. God was real to Richard, and the tension between God and Richard was as real as his frustration that he and I could not solve his problem with medications. In the framework of Alexander Leighton's work, Richard's religious sentiment was as real as his need for physical security.

I felt that I was in the same position as the friends of Job (the biblical character who was cursed by God with every imaginable affliction), trying to explain why this was happening to Richard yet helpless to relieve the suffering. I did not want to repeat the errors of Job's friends, for each of them gave apparently sage advice, yet the advice was of no value, and none of these friends remained by his side throughout his emotional suffering. I knew that maintaining our relationship was perhaps the most beneficial contribution I could make to Richard's problem.

I told Richard that I had no answer. My prayers for him were of no more value in relieving his depression than his own prayers. So I listened as Richard told me, time and again, of his complaint. "Why has God caused me this misery at the end of such a long and productive life? He could have taken me quickly when I suffered the heart attack. He could have let me die with dignity."

That answer puzzled me. I asked, "What do you mean by 'dignity'?"

He said he had become confused about relationships with God and humankind. He had lost confidence in his understanding about God and his ways in the world, and lost confidence that his own life made sense.

I confessed that I was confused as well. I was no better at predicting what God would do and why than Richard. I had the same fears he experienced. I also had no guarantee that my fate in the future would be any different from Richard's fate.

When I spoke of my own fears to Richard, I was stepping out of my comfort zone. I'm not one to reveal my fears to others, and I have as much desire to be in control as did Richard. Yet this confession to Richard seemed to change our relationship.

From then on I heard fewer comments from Richard about his anger with God. No answers came, but the questioning subsided, and Richard seemed much less frustrated. He spoke rarely of his tarnished image and more of the day-to-day struggles to maintain his functioning and the help he received from Tom. Still, he wished to see me regularly.

I saw Richard again one month after my confession. During the next four months he was too weak to make the trip to Durham. At the end of this four-month absence I stopped by his home while traveling to a professional meeting. We talked more as friends, companions on a long journey, than as doctor and patient. I suspected that visit would be the last time I would see Richard alive, and I suspected he sensed the same, though we parted as if we would be getting together soon in my office.

Two weeks later, Richard died while I was vacationing in Europe. I continue to see Tom, who has done well following Richard's death, especially as he found much support from the church. One of Richard's closest friends has taken Richard's former supportive role when Tom periodically experiences a crisis.

To this day I cannot accurately describe Richard as a "case." What I have written above does not do justice to what happened, nor to my feelings about the relationship, and certainly not to Richard's feelings. I do know, however, that Richard's relationship to his God and to his psychiatrist, a matter of the soul if you will, was the key to some type of resolution near the end of his life. I also know that Richard pressed me to the limit in my ability to understand his situation both as a psychiatrist and as a Christian. That is, I not only think about Richard as a person for whom I cared and respected, I think about him as a reminder of the difficult task I face in caring for persons experiencing severe emotional suffering.

Yet Richard does not leave me puzzled as do Jason, Barbara and Betty. Though I may not be able to express what happened, I am confident that we crossed a barrier together in our relationship as doctor and patient, a barrier for which neither psychiatry nor Christian counseling has no easy explanation. We engaged in a conversation that was therapeutic from a psychiatric perspective and that cut to the soul for both of us. For this reason Richard's story gives me confidence that a meaningful conversation—and at times debate—between psychiatry and Christianity can take us further along the road to healing the emotions.

Notes

Introduction

[1]The term *soul* is nebulous at best. I use the term in this book not as a theological or psychological construct but as an indication of the subjective experience of the person, and the recognition of that subjective experience by a therapist or other persons entering a helping relationship with those experiencing emotional suffering. A person doesn't *have* a soul but *is* soul—that is, "who I am in relationship with others and God." Therefore soul transcends the concepts of personality, self and identity. Despite what a therapist, or theologian for that matter, believes about the existence or nature of "God," a recognition of soul is a recognition of the subjective experience of the person not only in relationship with the world but also before God.

[2]Rainer Maria Rilke, *Letters to a Young Poet* (New York: W. W. Norton, 1934), pp. 57-58; emphasis mine.

[3]The descriptions of these persons have been modified so that they cannot be recognized (to maintain confidentiality) yet the elements of their stories are unchanged. I describe my interaction with these persons so that you, the reader, can share questions that I have not answered.

Chapter 1: Stories & Questions

[1]Paul Tournier, *The Meaning of Persons* (New York: Harper & Row, 1957).

[2]William Styron, *Darkness Visible: A Memoir of Madness* (New York: Random House, 1990).

[3]William Styron, *The Confessions of Nat Turner* (New York: Random House, 1966).

[4]Peter Kramer, *Listening to Prozac* (New York: Penguin, 1993).

[5]Melvin Konner, "Out of Darkness," *The New York Times Magazine,* October 2, 1994, pp. 70-73.

Chapter 2: Conversation & Debate

[1]I refer to severe emotional suffering throughout this book, yet I do not attempt to define this suffering explicitly. An explicit definition, as I discuss later, is one of the very trends

that undermine the soul of psychiatry. To provide more focus, however, I am not discussing the general angst of society, as, for example, described in W. H. Auden's long poem "The Age of Anxiety." Rather, I refer to the extraordinarily painful and alienated feelings that afflict a minority of persons often for discrete periods of their lives. These feelings are well described by William Styron in *Darkness Visible: A Memoir of Madness:* "In depression . . . the pain is unrelenting. . . . One does not abandon, even briefly, one's bed of nails, but is attached to it wherever one goes. . . . The situation of the walking wounded . . . the sufferer from depression . . . finds himself, like a walking casualty of war, thrust into the most intolerable social and family situations. There he must, despite the anguish devouring his brain, present a face approximating the one that is associated with ordinary events and companionship" ([New York: Random House, 1990], pp. 62-63).

[2]St. Augustine, *Confessions,* trans. E. B. Pusey (New York: Modern Library, 1949), pp. 166-87.

[3]Robert Burton, *The Anatomy of Melancholy,* ed. Floyd Dell and Paul Jordan-Smith (New York: Tudor, 1927), p. 8.

[4]Ibid., p. 100.

[5]F. G. Alexander and S. T. Selesnick, *The History of Psychiatry: An Evaluation of Psychiatric Thought and Practice from Prehistoric Times to the Present* (New York: New American Library, 1966).

[6]Ibid., p.140

[7]E. Brooks Holifield, *A History of Pastoral Care in America* (Nashville: Abingdon, 1983), p. 15.

[8]William Perkins, *The Whole Treatise of the Cases of Conscience,* ed. Thomas Merrill; William Perkins (1558-1602), Nieuwkoolp, Netherlands, 1966, as quoted in Holifield, *History of Pastoral Care,* p. 27.

[9]Thomas Szasz, *The Myth of Mental Illness* (New York: Harper & Row, 1974).

[10]Jane Murphy, "Psychiatric Labeling in Cross-Cultural Perspective," *Science* 191 (1976): 1019.

[11]Jose Barchilon's introduction to *Michel Foucault: Madness in Civilization,* trans. Richard Howard (New York: Vintage, 1965), pp. v-viii.

[12]Stanley Jackson, *Melancholia and Depression: From Hipprocratic Times to Modern Times* (New Haven, Conn.: Yale University Press, 1986), p. 328.

[13]Holifield, *History of Pastoral Care,* pp. 70-71.

[14]Alexander and Selesnick, *History of Psychiatry,* p. 151.

[15]Ibid., p. 152.

[16]*Diagnostic and Statistical Manual of Mental Disorders* (DSM-III, DSM-IIIR, DSM-IV; Washington, D.C.: American Psychiatric Association, 1980, 1987, 1994).

[17]Alexander and Selesnick, *History of Psychiatry,* pp. 212-13.

[18]Ibid., p. 213.

[19]Ibid., p. 173.

[20]William James, *The Varieties of Religious Experience: A Study in Human Nature*

(Cambridge, Mass.: Harvard University Press, 1902).

[21] Auguste Comte, *A General View of Positivism,* trans. J. H. Bridges (New York: Robert Speller & Sons, 1975).

[22] John Bunyan, *Pilgrim's Progress* (1678; reprint New York: Dodd, Mead, 1909).

[23] David M. Wulff, *Psychology of Religion: Classic and Contemporary Views* (New York: John Wiley & Sons, 1991).

[24] Ibid., p. 271.

[25] Ibid., p. 272; Ernest Jones, *The Life and Work of Sigmund Freud,* vol. 3, *The Last Phase* (New York: Basic Books, 1957), p. 20; Heinrich Meng and Ernst Freud, *Psychoanalysis and Faith: The Letters of Sigmund Freud and Oskar Pfister,* trans. Eric Mosbacher (New York: Basic Books, 1963), p. 63.

[26] Peter Gay, *Freud: A Life for Our Time* (New York: Doubleday, 1988), pp. 617-18.

[27] Ibid., pp. 11-12.

[28] Ludwig Buchner, *Kraft und Stoff: Empirisch-Naturphilosophische Studien* (Leipsig: 1855); as discussed in Hans Küng, *Freud and the Problem of God,* trans. Edward Guinn (New Haven, Conn.: Yale University Press, 1979), pp. 5-6.

[29] Ludwig Feuerbach, *The Essence of Christianity,* ed. E. Graham Waring and F. W. Strothmann (New York: Frederick Unger, 1957).

[30] Sigmund Freud, *The Future of an Illusion* (1927), in *Standard Edition of the Complete Psychological Works of Sigmund Freud* (24 vols.), ed. J. Strachey (London: Hogarth/Institute of Psycho-analysis, 1953-1964), pp. 1-156.

[31] Sigmund Freud, *The Psychopathology of Everyday Life,* in *Standard Edition,* 6:258-59.

[32] Sigmund Freud, *Leonardo da Vinci and a Memory of His Childhood,* in *Standard Edition,* 11:57-137.

[33] Floyd Westendorp, "The Value of Freud's Illusion," *Journal of Psychology and Theology* 3 (1975): 82-89.

[34] Carl G. Jung, *The Integration of Personality* (New York: Farrar & Reinhart, 1939); Carl G. Jung, *The Structure and Dynamics of the Psyche,* vol. 8 of *The Collected Works* (New York: Pantheon, 1960); John D. Carter, "Personality and Christian Maturity: A Process Congruity Model," *Journal of Psychology and Theology* 2 (1974): 190-201.

[35] Wulff, *Psychology of Religion,* pp. 432-33.

[36] Carl G. Jung, *Psychotherapists or the Clergy,* vol. 11 of *Collected Works,* 2nd ed. (Princeton, N.J.: Princeton University Press, 1932), p. 334.

[37] Heinrich Meng and Anna Freud, *Psychoanalysis and Faith* (New York: Basic Books, 1963); Westendorp, "Value of Freud's Illusion."

[38] Meng and Freud, *Psychoanalysis and Faith,* p. 127.

[39] Westendorp, "Value of Freud's Illusion," pp. 82-89.

[40] Gregory Zilboorg, *Psychoanalysis and Religion* (New York: Farrar, Straus & Cudahy, 1962); Küng, *Freud and the Problem of God* (New Haven, Conn.: Yale University Press, 1929).

[41] Zilboorg, *Psychoanalysis and Religion,* p. 97.

[42] Karl Menninger. *Whatever Became of Sin?* (New York: Hawthorn, 1973), p. 189.

[43]Ibid., p. 224.

[44]Thomas Jobe, "American Soul-Doctrine at the Turn of the Century: Toward the Psychiatry of the Spiritual," in *Religious and Ethical Factors in Psychiatric Practice,* ed. Don S. Browning, Thomas Jobe and Ian Evison (Chicago: Nelson-Hall, 1990), pp. 107-28.

[45]Paul Tillich, "You're Accepted" in *The Shaking of the Foundations* (New York: Charles Scribner's Sons, 1948) pp. 153-63.

[46]Don S. Browning, Thomas Jobe and Ian S. Evison, eds., *Religious and Ethical Factors in Psychiatric Practice* (Chicago: Nelson-Hall, 1990), p. 34.

[47]Paul Tillich, *The Theology of Culture* (New York: Oxford University Press, 1959).

[48]Paul Tillich, *The Courage to Be* (New Haven, Conn.: Yale University Press, 1952), pp. 52-53.

[49]Ibid., p. 52.

[50]Paul Tillich, *Systematic Theology* (Chicago: University of Chicago Press, 1951), 1:212; Browning, Jobe and Evison, *Religious and Ethical Factors,* p. 35.

[51]Browning, Jobe and Evison, *Religious and Ethical Factors,* p. 30; Reinhold Niebuhr, *Beyond Tragedy* (New York: Charles Scribner's, 1937).

[52]Reinhold Niebuhr, *Moral Man and Immoral Society* (New York: Charles Scribner's Sons, 1932), p. xi.

[53]Reinhold Niebuhr, "Human Creativity and Self-Concern in Freud's Thoughts," in *Freud and the Twentieth Century,* ed. Benjamin Nelson (Gloucester, U.K.: Peter Smith, 1974), p. 269; Browning, Jobe and Evison, *Religious and Ethical Factors,* p. 31.

[54]Reinhold Niebuhr, *The Nature and Destiny of Man* (New York: Charles Scribner's Sons, 1941), 1:43.

[55]Ibid., p. 42; Browning, Jobe and Evison, *Religious and Ethical Factors,* p. 31.

[56]Browning, Jobe and Evison, *Religious and Ethical Factors,* p. 32.

[57]H. Richard Niebuhr, "A Story of Our Life," in *The Meaning of Revelation* (New York: Macmillan, 1941), pp. 43-81.

[58]Robert Burns, "To a Louse" (1786).

[59]Niebuhr, "Story of Our Life," p. 43.

[60]Arnold Cooper, Allen Frances and Michael Sacks, "The Psychoanalytic Model," in *Psychiatry,* ed. R. Michels et al. (Philadelphia: Lippincott, 1990), 1:11.

[61]Browning, Jobe and Evison, *Religious and Ethical Factors,* pp. 19-20, 34-38; Paul Ricoeur, *Freud and Philosophy* (New Haven, Conn.: Yale University Press, 1970).

[62]Ricoeur, *Freud and Philosophy,* p. 8.

[63]Wulff, *Psychology of Religion,* pp. 303-4.

[64]Ricoeur, *Freud and Philosophy,* p. 4.

[65]Holifield, *History of Pastoral Care,* pp. 244-46.

[66]Anton Boisen, *The Exploration of the Inner World* (New York: Harper & Row, 1936), pp. 266-67, as quoted in Howard J. Clinebell, *Basic Types of Pastoral Counseling* (Nashville: Abingdon, 1966), p. 276.

[67]Clinebell, *Basic Types,* p. 28.

[68]Paul Tillich, *The Religious Situation,* trans. H. Richard Niebuhr (New York: Meridian,

1932), as described in Holifield, *History of Pastoral Care,* p. 250.

[69]Rollo May, *The Springs of Creative Living: A Study of Human Nature and God* (Nashville: Abingdon, 1939), as described in Holifield, *History of Pastoral Care,* pp. 251-53.

[70]Holifield, *History of Pastoral Care,* p. 259.

[71]William Glasser, *The Identity Society* (New York: Harper & Row, 1972).

[72]Holifield, *History of Pastoral Care,* p. 262.

[73]Erich Fromm, *Man for Himself* (New York: Rinehart, 1947); Erich Fromm, *The Art of Loving* (New York: Harper & Row, 1956), as described in Holifield, *History of Pastoral Care,* pp. 283-85.

[74]Holifield, *History of Pastoral Care,* pp. 295-98.

[75]Ibid., p. 300. See reference in Holifield for extensive documentation of the debate between Niebuhr and Rogers.

[76]Ibid., p. 311.

[77]Albert Outler, *Psychotherapy and the Christian Message* (New York: Harper, 1954).

[78]Holifield, *History of Pastoral Care,* p. 347.

[79]A. T. Grounds, "Lectures on Heaven: An excursion into the Playground of the Theologies," *British Medical Journal* 283 (1981): 2664, as quoted in Robert Sevensky, "Religion, Psychology and Mental Health," *American Journal of Psychotherapy* 38 (1984): 73.

[80]John D. Carter, "Secular and Sacred Models of Psychology in Religion," *Journal of Psychology and Theology* 5 (1977): 197-208.

[81]Feuerbach, *Essence of Christianity,* p. 65.

[82]Earl Biddle, *Integration of Psychiatry and Religion* (New York: Collier, 1955).

[83]Ibid., p. 8.

[84]Edgar Draper et al., "On the Diagnostic Value of Religious Ideation," *Archives of General Psychiatry* 13 (1965): 202-7.

[85]Carl Christensen, "Religious Conversion," *Archives of General Psychiatry* 9 (1963): 207-16.

[86]Stephen Carter, *The Culture of Disbelief* (New York: BasicBooks, 1992).

[87]H. E. Kagan, *Psychiatry and Religion* (Cleveland, Ohio: Minnie K. Lansberg Memorial Foundation, 1952), as quoted in Kenneth Appel, "Psychiatry and Religion," in *American Handbook of Psychiatry,* ed. Silvaro Arieti (New York: Basic Books, 1974), 1:993.

[88]O. Hobart Mowrer, *The Crisis in Psychiatry and Religion* (Princeton, N.J.: Van Nostrand, 1961), p. 60.

[89]Jay E. Adams, *Competent to Counsel* (Grand Rapids: Baker Book House, 1970), p. xvii.

[90]Ibid.

[91]A series of recent publications that have been widely distributed by the International Association of Scientologists through a group called the Citizens Commission on Human Rights is blatantly antipsychiatry. Titles of these publications include "Psychiatry Destroying Religion" and "Psychiatry—the Ultimate Betrayal." The focus of these attacks is psychiatry as it was practiced at midcentury. Freud therefore is their most frequent target.

[92]Küng, *Freud and the Problem of God.*

[93] Appel, "Psychiatry and Religion," p. 992.

[94] Viktor Frankl, *The Doctor and the Soul: From Psychotherapy to Logotherapy* (New York: Alfred A. Knopf, 1955); Erik Erikson, *Childhood and Society* (New York: W. W. Norton, 1950); Rollo May, *Man's Search for Himself* (New York: W. W. Norton, 1953).

[95] Stanley Hauerwas, *A Community of Character: Toward a Self-Constructive Christian Social Ethic* (Notre Dame, Ind.: University of Notre Dame Press, 1981).

[96] Sigmund Freud, *Totem and Taboo: Some Points of Agreement Between the Mental Lives of Savages and Neurotics,* in *Standard Edition,* 13:1-161.

[97] Ibid., 13:141-42.

[98] Karl Marx, *Critique of the Helegian Philosophy of Right* (1844), as quoted in John Bartlett, *Familiar Quotations* (Boston: Little, Brown and Company, 1980), p. 562.

[99] Sigmund Freud, *The Future of an Illusion,* in *Standard Edition,* 21:17-18.

[100] Steven J. Gould, interview in *Raleigh News and Observer,* April 7, 1994.

[101] Gary Collins, *Christian Counseling: A Comprehensive Guide* (Waco, Tex.: Word, 1980), pp. 86, 91-92.

[102] Albert Camus, *The Myth of Sisyphus,* trans. Justin O'Brien (London: Penguin, 1975), p. 11.

[103] *Diagnostic and Statistical Manual of Mental Disorders,* 4th ed. (DSM-IV).

[104] Lillian H. Robinson, ed., *Psychiatry and Religion: Overlapping Concerns* (Washington, D.C.: American Psychiatric Press, 1986); J. Roland Fleck and John D. Carter, *Psychology and Christianity: Integrative Readings* (Nashville: Abingdon, 1981).

[105] Roy H. Hart, "Psychiatry and Religion: We Need More Than Rapprochement," *Psychiatric News,* May 20, 1994.

[106] Sharon Begley, "One Pill Makes You Larger, and One Pill Makes You Smaller . . ." *Newsweek,* February 7, 1994, pp. 37-43.

Chapter 3: Psychiatry Loses Its Soul

[1] Vance Packard, *The Hidden Persuaders* (New York: David McKay, 1957).

[2] Martin Gross, *The Psychological Society* (New York: Random House, 1978).

[3] Franz Alexander and T. M. French, *Studies in Psychosomatic Medicine* (New York: Ronald, 1948).

[4] Jerry Foder, "The Mind-Brain Problem," *Scientific American* 244 (1981): 114-23; Donald Mender, *The Myth of Neuropsychiatry* (New York: Plenum, 1994), p. 38.

[5] Silvano Arieti, *Interpretation of Schizophrenia* (New York: Basic Books, 1974).

[6] Hannah Greene, *I Never Promised You a Rose Garden* (New York: Holt, Rinehart and Winston, 1969).

[7] Frieda Fromm-Reichmann, *Principles of Intensive Psychotherapy* (Chicago: University of Chicago Press, 1950), as described in Franz Alexander and Sheldon Selesnick, *The History of Psychiatry* (New York: Mentor, 1966), p. 406.

[8] Melvin Sabshin, "Turning Points in Twentieth-Century American Psychiatry," *American Journal of Psychiatry* 147 (1990): 1267-74.

[9] Nathan Ackerman, *The Psychodynamics of Family Life* (New York: Basic Books, 1958);

Eric Berne, *Games People Play* (New York: Grove, 1964).

[10]George Mora, "Historical and Theoretical Trends in Psychiatry," in *Comprehensive Textbook of Psychiatry,* 3rd ed., ed. Harold Kaplan, Alfred Freedmann and Benjamin Sadock (Baltimore: Williams and Wilkins, 1980), pp. 4-98.

[11]Thomas S. Szasz, *The Myth of Mental Illness* (New York: Harper & Row, 1961).

[12]Ibid., p. 262.

[13]Jay E. Adams, *Competent to Counsel* (Grand Rapids, Mich.: Baker Book House, 1970).

[14]Michel Foucault, *Madness and Civilization,* trans. Richard Howard (New York: Vintage, 1965).

[15]E. Fuller Torey, *The Mind Game: Witch Doctors and Psychiatrists* (New York: Emerson Hall, 1972).

[16]Hannah H. Decker, *Freud, Dora and Vienna, 1900* (New York: Free Press, 1991).

[17]Sabshin, "Turning Points," p. 1271.

[18]F. Adams, *The Genuine Works of Hippocrates* (Baltimore: Williams and Wilkins, 1939), p. 366; Michael R. Tremble, *Biological Psychiatry* (New York: John Wiley & Sons, 1988), p. 1.

[19]Paul Churchland, *The Engine of Reason, the Seat of the Soul* (Cambridge, Mass.: M.I.T. Press, 1994); Daniel Dennett, *Cousciousness Explained* (New York: Little, Brown, 1991).

[20]Peter Kramer, *Listening to Prozac* (New York: Penguin, 1993).

[21]Sharon Begley, "One Pill Makes You Larger, and One Makes You Smaller . . ." *Newsweek,* February 7, 1994, pp. 37-43.

[22]David Wulff, *Psychology of Religion* (New York: John Wiley, 1991), p. 54.

[23]Robert Burton, *The Anatomy of Melancholia* (New York: Tudor, 1938), p. 968.

[24]Wulff, p. 42; G. Stanley Hall, *Adolescence: Its Psychology and Its Relation to Physiology, Anthropology, Sociology, Sex, Crime, Religion and Education* (New York: D. Appleton, 1904), pp. 295-301.

[25]G. Stanley Hall, *Life and Confessions of a Psychologist* (New York: D. Appleton, 1923), p. 574; Wulff, *Psychology of Religion,* p. 43.

[26]Arnold J. Mandell, "Toward a Psychobiology of Transcendent: God in the Brain," paper presented at the Emergent Brain Properties symposium at the Eleventh Annual Winter Conference on Brain Research, Keystone, Colorado, January 1978.

[27]F. J. Hacker, *Crusaders, Criminals and Crazies* (New York: Bantam, 1978); William Sargant, *Battle for the Mind: Physiology of Conversion and Brain-washing* (London: Heinemann, 1957); George A. Sheehan, *Advice and Philosophy for Runners* (New York: Simon & Schuster, 1978).

[28]Edward O. Wilson, *On Human Nature* (Cambridge, Mass.: Harvard University Press, 1978), p. 192.

[29]Ernst Mayr, *Toward a New Philosophy of Biology: Observations of an Evolutionist* (Cambridge, Mass.: Harvard University Press, 1988), p. 82.

[30]Ibid., p. 83.

[31]Edward Hundert, *Philosophy, Psychiatry and Neuroscience: A Synthetic Analysis of the Varieties of Human Experience* (New York: Oxford University Press, 1989).

[32]Arnold M. Cooper, "Will Neuropsychiatry Influence Psychoanalysis?" *American Journal of Psychiatry* 142 (1985): 1395-402.

[33]Sabshin, "Turning Points," p. 1274.

[34]Kramer, *Listening to Prozac,* p. 300.

[35]Ibid.

[36]Ibid.

[37]Begley, "One Pill Makes You Larger," p. 42.

[38]Aldous Huxley, *Brave New World* (New York: Harper & Brothers, 1932), pp. 170-71.

[39]José Ortega y Gasset, *The Revolt of the Masses* (New York: W. W. Norton, 1932).

[40]Ibid., p. 114.

[41]*Diagnostic and Statistical Manual of Mental Disorders,* 3rd ed. (DSM-III; Washington, D.C.: American Psychiatric Association, 1980).

[42]*Diagnostic and Statistical Manual of Mental Disorders,* 3rd ed. rev. (DSM-IIIR; Washington, D.C.: American Psychiatric Association, 1987); *Diagnostic and Statistical Manual of Mental Disorders,* 4th ed. (DSM-IV; Washington, D.C.: American Psychiatric Association, 1994).

[43]Percy W. Bridgman, *The Logic of Modern Physics* (New York: Macmillan, 1948).

[44]DSM-IV.

[45]David Lukoff, Francis Lu and Robert Turner, "Toward a More Culturally Sensitive DSM-IV: Psycho-religious and Psycho-spiritual Problems," *The Journal of Nervous and Mental Diseases* 180 (1992): 673-82.

[46]David Larson, a psychiatrist, committed evangelical Christian and friend, exemplifies this approach. He and his wife, Susan, wrote *The Forgotten Factor in Physical and Mental Health: What Does the Research Show?* (Arlington, Va.: National Institute for Healthcare Research, 1992), the forgotten factor being religion. I suspect they are correct that self-reports of religious beliefs are associated with a lower frequency of mental illness. Yet I am not certain if this association stimulates meaningful conversation between psychiatrists and Christians any more than if religious beliefs were positively associated with mental illness. At best, the identification encourages psychiatrists and Christians to sit at the same table and begin the conversation. For this reason I have coauthored many papers with Dr. Larson; these data do challenge the perception that religion encourages mental stress. At worst, however, I believe the statistical association *becomes* the conversation.

[47]Franz Alexander and Sheldon Selesnick, *The History of Psychiatry* (New York: New American Library, 1966), pp. 328-30.

[48]Alexander Lief, *The Common Sense Psychiatry of Adolf Meyer* (New York: McGraw-Hill, 1943), p. x.

[49]Aaron T. Beck, *Cognitive Therapy and the Emotional Disorder* (New York: International University Press, 1976).

[50]Ibid., p. 17.

[51]Anthony Burgess, *A Clockwork Orange* (New York: Ballantine, 1962).

[52]B. F. Skinner, *Walden II* (New York: Macmillan, 1948).

[53]Gerald L. Klerman et al., *Interpersonal Psychotherapy of Depression* (New York: Basic Books, 1984).

[54]Arthur Kleinman, *Rethinking Psychiatry: From Cultural Category to Personal Experience* (New York: Free Press, 1988).

[55]Ibid., pp. 132-33.

[56]Harold Bloom, *The American Religion: The Emergence of a Post-Christian Nation* (New York: Simon & Schuster, 1992), p. 257.

[57]David D. Burns, *Feeling Good: The New Mood Therapy* (New York: Signet, 1981). The back cover of Burns's book, which describes cognitive therapy for the public, reads: "You feel the way you think. . . . This book . . . outlines a systematic program for controlling thought distortions . . . and achieving a life rich in strength, self-assurance, and accomplishment." Is it any wonder that the commonsense therapy of Aaron Beck appeals to the religious in the United States?

[58]Kleinman, *Rethinking Psychiatry,* p. 132.

[59]Ibid., p. 133.

[60]Thomas A. Harris, *I'm OK, You're OK: A Practical Guide to Transactional Analysis* (New York: Harper & Row, 1967).

[61]Thomas Moore, *Care of the Soul: A Guide for Cultivating Depth and Sacredness in Everyday Life* (New York: Harper, 1992), pp. xi-xii.

[62]Jeffrey H. Boyd, *Soul Psychology* (Cheshire, U.K.: Soul Research Institute, 1994), p. 47.

Chapter 4: Christianity Loses Its Mind

[1]Sydney E. Ahlstrom, *A Religious History of the American People* (New Haven, Conn.: Yale University Press, 1972), p. 1080.

[2]Richard Coleman, *Issues of Theological Warfare: Evangelicals and Liberals* (Grand Rapids, Mich.: Eerdmans, 1972).

[3]Ahlstrom, *Religious History,* p. 909.

[4]Ronald Numbers, *The Creationists: The Evolution of Scientific Creationism* (Berkeley: University of California Press, 1992).

[5]Ahlstrom, *Religious History,* p. 912.

[6]Ibid., p. 913.

[7]H. L. Mencken, "Protestantism and the Republic," in *Prejudices,* ed. Wilber C. Abbot (New York: Alfred A. Knopf, 1926), pp. 104-5, 115; as quoted in Ahlstrom, *Religious History,* pp. 915-16.

[8]Ahlstrom, *Religious History,* p. 915.

[9]Mark A. Noll, *The Scandal of the Evangelical Mind* (Grand Rapids, Mich.: Eerdmans, 1994).

[10]J. I. Packer, *Fundamentalism and the Word of God* (London: Inter-Varsity Fellowship, 1958), p. 9.

[11]Carl F. H. Henry, *The Uneasy Conscience of Modern Fundamentalism* (Grand Rapids, Mich.: Eerdmans, 1947), as quoted in Coleman, *Issues of Theological Warfare,* p. 25.

[12]Billy Graham, interview, *Christianity Today,* November 7, 1969, p. 34; as quoted in

Coleman, *Issues of Theological Warfare,* p. 26.

[13]Ahlstrom, *Religious History,* p. 959.

[14]Harold Bloom, *The American Religion: The Emergence of a Post-Christian Nation* (New York: Simon & Schuster, 1992).

[15]Robert N. Bellah et al., *Habits of the Heart: Individualism and Commitment in American Life* (Berkeley: University of California Press, 1985), p. 235.

[16]Bloom, *American Religion,* p. 219.

[17]Paul Tournier, *The Doctor's Case Book in Light of the Bible,* trans. Edwin Hudson (New York: Harper & Row, 1954); Paul Tournier, *The Meaning of Persons,* trans. Edwin Hudson (New York: Harper & Row, 1957).

[18]Tournier, *Meaning of Persons,* pp. 118-19.

[19]Ibid., p. 233.

[20]Tournier, *Doctor's Case Book,* p. 39.

[21]Albert Outler, *Psychotherapy and the Christian Message* (New York: Harper & Row, 1954).

[22]Ibid., p. 8.

[23]Ibid., pp. 7-8.

[24]Ibid., p. 244.

[25]Ibid., p. 247.

[26]Ibid., p. 255.

[27]Ibid., p. 257.

[28]Norman Vincent Peale, *The Power of Positive Thinking* (New York: Prentice-Hall, 1952).

[29]Tim LaHaye, *How to Win over Depression* (Grand Rapids, Mich.: Zondervan, 1974).

[30]James D. Mallory Jr., *The Kink and I: A Psychiatrist's Guide to Untwisted Living* (Wheaton, Ill.: Victor, 1973).

[31]Gary Collins, "Popular Christian Psychologies: Some Reflections," *Journal of Psychology and Theology* 3 (1975): 127-32.

[32]John D. Carter, "The Psychology of Gothard and Basic Youth Conflict Seminar," *Journal of Psychology and Theology* 2 (1975): 249-59.

[33]Eric Berne, *Games People Play* (New York: Grove, 1964); Frederick S. Perls, *Gestalt Therapy Verbatim* (New York: Bantam, 1970); Carl R. Rogers, *On Becoming a Person* (Boston: Houghton Mifflin, 1961).

[34]Bruce Larson, *Living on the Growing Edge* (Grand Rapids, Mich.: Zondervan, 1968).

[35]Viktor Frankl, *Man's Search for Meaning* (New York: Beacon, 1963). Larson reduces Frankl's writings to a level that can be understood by a person with a high-school education. He focuses on problems that pervade most of humankind, not the more severe emotional problems, and calls upon Scripture frequently. Though he references Christian theologians such as Dietrich Bonhoeffer and non-Christian psychiatrists such as Frankl, he provides no reference or bibliography for their writings, something that would be anathema to the academy. In other words, Larson attempts to avoid giving the appearance of an academic, one of Collins's characteristics of a popular Christian counselor.

[36]Larson, *Living on the Growing Edge,* p. 42.

[37]Ibid.

[38]LaHaye, introduction to *How to Win over Depression.*

[39]Ibid.

[40]Ibid.

[41]LaHaye, *How to Win over Depression,* pp. 200-206.

[42]David Seamands, *Healing for Damaged Emotions* (Wheaton, Ill.: Victor, 1983), p. 8.

[43]Ibid., p. 65.

[44]Ibid.

[45]Joseph Wolpe, *Psychotherapy by Reciprocal Inhibitions* (Palo Alto, Calif.: Stanford University Press, 1958).

[46]Bernie S. Siegel, *Love, Medicine and Miracles* (New York: Harper & Row, 1986).

[47]Ibid., p. 4.

[48]Ibid., p. 152.

[49]Robert Schuller, *Tough Times Never Last, but Tough People Do!* (Nashville: Thomas Nelson, 1983), pp. 9-10.

[50]George Marsden, *Reforming Fundamentalism: Fuller Seminary and the New Evangelicalism* (Grand Rapids, Mich.: Eerdmans, 1987), p. 233.

[51]Ibid.

[52]Ibid., p. 234.

[53]Ibid.

[54]William P. Wilson, *The Grace to Grow: The Power of Christian Faith in Emotional Healing* (Waco, Tex.: Word, 1984).

[55]E. Mansell Pattison, "Social and Psychological Aspects of Religion in Psychotherapy," *Journal of Nervous and Mental Diseases* 141 (1966): 586-96.

[56]Directory of the Psychiatry Section of the Christian Medical Society, 1985.

[57]Hendrika Vande Kemp and H. Newton Malony, *Psychology and Theology in Western Thought (1672-1965): A Historical and Annotated Bibliography* (Millwood, N.Y.: Kraus International, 1984).

[58]Wilson, *Grace to Grow,* pp. 87, 93.

[59]Promotional brochure, New Life Centers, 1995.

[60]Tim Stafford, "Franchising Hope," *Christianity Today,* May 18, 1992, pp. 22-26.

[61]Phillip Guerin, "Family Therapy: The First Twenty-five Years," in *Family Therapy: Theory and Practice,* ed. Phillip Guerin (New York: Gardner, 1976), pp. 2-22.

[62]Nathan Ackerman, "The Family as a Social and Emotional Unit," *Bulletin of the Kansas Mental Hygiene Society,* 1937.

[63]James Dobson, *Dare to Discipline* (Wheaton, Ill.: Tyndale House, 1970).

[64]Haim Ginott, *Between Parent and Child: New Solutions to Old Problems* (New York: Avon, 1965).

[65]Dobson, *Dare to Discipline,* pp. 13-14.

[66]Ibid., p. 69.

[67]James Davison Hunter, *Culture Wars: The Struggle to Define America* (New York: BasicBooks, 1991), p. 64.

[68]C. W. Socaides, *The Overt Homosexual* (New York: Grune and Stratton, 1968); Ervin Bieber, *Homosexuality: A Psychoanalytic Study* (New York: Basic Books, 1962).

[69]*Psychiatric News,* April 15, 1994, p. 18.

[70]Memorandum from Russell Brubaker and Richard Heckmann to all psychiatry section members re upcoming vote on homosexuality and abortion, dated May 2, 1994.

[71]Stephen L. Carter, *The Culture of Disbelief* (New York: BasicBooks, 1993), p. 4.

Chapter 5: Filling the Vacuum

[1]Reynolds Price, *A Whole New Life: An Illness and a Healing* (New York: Atheneum, 1994), pp. 49-50.

[2]Donald A. Schon, *The Reflective Practitioner: How Professionals Think in Action* (New York: Basic Books, 1983).

[3]Margaret Gerteis et al., "Medicine and Health from the Patient's Perspective," in *Through the Patient's Eyes: Understanding and Promoting Patient-Centered Care,* ed. Margaret Gerteis et al. (San Francisco: Jossey-Bass, 1993), pp. 1-18.

[4]Ibid., p. 6.

[5]Eric Cassel, *The Nature of Suffering and the Goals of Medicine* (New York: Oxford University Press, 1991), p. vii.

[6]Arthur Kleinman, *The Illness Narratives: Suffering and the Human Condition* (New York: BasicBooks, 1988).

[7]Ibid., pp. xiii-xiv.

[8]Patricia Churchland, *Neurophilosophy: Toward a Unified Science of the Mind-Brain* (Cambridge, Mass.: M.I.T. Press, 1986), p. ix.

[9]"In Search of the Sacred," *Newsweek,* November 28, 1994, p. 53.

[10]George Marsden, *Religion and American Culture* (New York: Harcourt Brace Jovanovich, 1990), p. 254.

[11]Harold Bloom, *The American Religion: The Emergence of the Post-Christian Nation* (New York: Simon & Schuster, 1992), pp. 181-88.

[12]Ibid., p. 184.

[13]Thomas Moore, *Care of the Soul: A Guide for Cultivating Depth and Sacredness in Everyday Life* (New York: Harper, 1992).

[14]Ibid., p. 137.

[15]Ibid., p. 203.

[16]M. Scott Peck, *The Road Less Traveled: The New Psychology of Love, Traditional Values and Spiritual Growth* (New York: Simon & Schuster, 1978).

[17]Ibid., pp. 11-12.

[18]Ibid., p. 185.

[19]Ibid., p. 186.

[20]Ibid., p. 69.

[21]Irving D. Yalom, *Existential Psychotherapy* (New York: Basic Books, 1980).

[22]Ibid., pp. 4-5.

[23]Ludwig Binswanger, "Freud's Conception of Man in Light of Anthropology," in *Being*

in the World, trans. Jacob Needleman (New York: Harper & Row, 1963); Ludwig Binswanger, "The Case of Ellen West: An Anthropological-Clinical Study," *Schweizer Archiv fur Neurologie und Psychiatrie* 53 (1945): 255-77; Dieter Wyss, *Psychoanalytic Schools from the Beginning to the Present,* trans. Gerald Onn (New York: Jason Aronson, 1973), pp. 384-404.

[24]Wyss, *Psychoanalytic Schools,* p. 395.

[25]Yalom, *Existential Psychotherapy,* p. 355.

[26]Ibid., p. 401.

[27]Ibid., p. 355

[28]Ibid.

[29]Ibid., p. 482.

[30]Ibid., p. 45-46.

[31]Robert Coles, *The Spiritual Life of Children* (Boston: Houghton Mifflin, 1990), p. xvi.

[32]A. E. Bergin, "Psychotherapy and Religious Values," *Journal of Consulting and Clinical Psychology* 48 (1980): 95-105.

[33]Albert Ellis, "Psychotherapy and Atheistic Values: A Response to A. E. Bergin's 'Psychotherapy in Religious Values,' " *Journal of Consulting in Clinical Psychology* 48 (1980): 635-39.

[34]A. E. Bergin, "Values and Religious Issues in Psychotherapy and Mental Health," *American Psychologist* 46 (1991): 394-403; A. E. Bergin and J. B. Jensen, "Religiosity of Psychotherapist: A National Survey," *Psychotherapy* 27 (1990): 3-7.

[35]A. E. Bergin, "Religiosity and Mental Health: A Critical Reevaluation and Meta-analysis," *Professional Psychology: Research in Practice* 14 (1983): 170-81.

[36]Di Stubbs and Ben Finny, "The Samaritans," paper presented at Research into Aging meeting, London, November 12, 1994.

[37]Stanley Hauerwas and L. Gregory Jones, *Why Narrative? Readings in Narrative Theology* (Grand Rapids, Mich.: Eerdmans, 1989).

[38]Stanley Hauerwas, *A Community of Care: Toward a Constructive Christian Social Ethic* (Notre Dame, Ind.: University of Notre Dame Press, 1981), p. 144.

[39]H. Richard Niebuhr, *The Meaning of Revelation* (New York: Macmillan, 1941), p. 45.

[40]Hauerwas, *Community of Care,* p. 127.

[41]Stanley Hauerwas and David Burrell, "From System to Story: An Alternative Pattern for Rationality in Ethics," in *Truthfulness and Tragedy: Further Investigation in Christian Ethics,* ed. Stanley Hauerwas (Notre Dame, Ind.: University of Notre Dame Press, 1977), pp. 15-39.

[42]Joseph English, in *Psychiatric News,* November 4, 1994, p. 8.

Chapter 6: The Care of Souls & Minds

[1]Sigmund Freud, *Civilization and Its Discontents,* 21:57-145; *Moses and Monotheism: Three Essays,* 23:7-137; *Totem and Taboo,* 13:1-161; all in *Standard Edition of the Complete Works of Sigmund Freud,* ed. J. Strachey, 24 vols. (London: Hogarth, 1953-1974); C. S. Lewis, *Mere Christianity* (New York: Macmillan, 1952); C. S. Lewis,

Miracles (New York: Macmillan, 1947); C. S. Lewis, *The Problem of Pain* (New York: Macmillan, 1962).

[2]Bruce Lawrence, *Defenders of God* (New York: Harper & Row, 1989), pp. 61-62.

[3]Paul Tillich, *Systematic Theology,* 3 vols. (Chicago: University of Chicago Press, 1976); Paul Tillich, *On Art and Architecture,* ed. John Dillenberger and Jane Dillenberger (New York: Crossroad, 1987).

[4]Clifford Geertz, *The Interpretation of Cultures* (New York: Basic Books, 1973), pp. 87-88.

[5]Edward M. Hundert, *Philosophy, Psychiatry and Neuroscience: Three Approaches to the Mind* (Oxford: Oxford University Press, 1989); Leston Havens, *Approaches to the Mind: Movement of Psychiatric Schools from Sects Toward Science* (Boston: Little, Brown, 1973).

[6]Robert N. Wilson, "Continuities in Social Psychiatry," in *Further Explorations in Social Psychiatry,* ed. Berton H. Kaplan, Robert N. Wilson and Alexander H. Leighton (New York: Basic Books, 1976), p. 7.

[7]Jean-Jacques Rousseau, *A Discourse on the Origin of Inequality,* trans. G. D. H. Cole (New York: Everyman Library, 1964).

[8]St. Anselm, *The Proslogion,* trans. Sister Benedicta Ward (New York: Penguin, 1973).

[9]Alexander Leighton, *My Name Is Legion* (New York: Basic Books, 1951), p. 232.

[10]Ibid., p. 148.

[11]Edward M. Hundert, *Lessons from an Optical Illusion: On Nature and Nurture, Knowledge and Values* (Cambridge, Mass.: Harvard University Press, 1995), pp. 184-97.

[12]Alasdair MacIntyre, *After Virtue,* 2nd ed. (Notre Dame, Ind.: University of Notre Dame Press, 1984).

[13]Leighton, *My Name Is Legion,* p. 228.

[14]Martin L. Gross, *The Psychological Society* (New York: Random House, 1978), pp. 3-4.

[15]James Davison Hunter, *Culture Wars: The Struggle to Define America* (New York: BasicBooks, 1991).

[16]Ibid., p. 43.

[17]Stanley Hauerwas and William H. Willimon, *Resident Aliens* (Nashville: Abingdon, 1989), pp. 11-12.

[18]Ibid., pp. 12-13.

[19]MacIntyre, *After Virtue,* p. 263.

[20]Alasdair MacIntyre, *Whose Justice? Which Rationality?* (Notre Dame, Ind.: University of Notre Dame Press, 1988); Hunter, *Culture Wars,* pp. 315, 319.

[21]Hunter, *Culture Wars,* pp. 320-25.

[22]John T. McNeill, preface to *A History of the Cure of Souls* (New York: Harper & Brothers, 1951).

Index